Kombucha Rediscovered!

Klaus Kaufmann

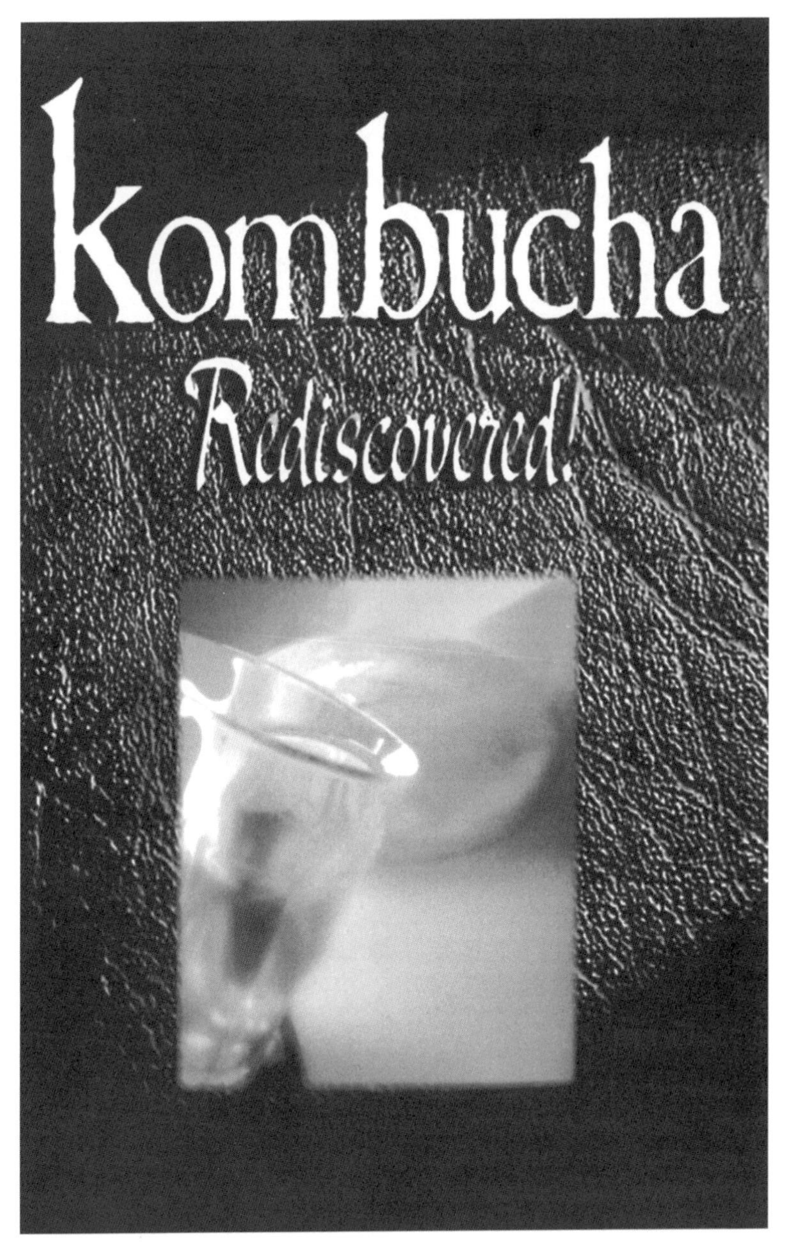

A Guide to the Medicinal Benefits of an Ancient Healing Tea

This book is informational only and should not be considered a substitute for consultation with a duly licensed medical doctor. Any attempt to diagnose or treat an illness should come under the direction of a physician. The author is not himself a medical doctor and does not purport to offer medical advice, make diagnoses, prescribe remedies for specific medical conditions or substitute for medical consultation.

Published by

Alive Books
PO Box 80055 Burnaby BC Canada V5H 3X1

Cover Design: Peter Virag
Typesetting/Layout: Peter Virag and Lisa Trommeshauser
Front Cover Photo: Ron Crompton
Back Cover Photo: Ron Crompton

First Printing - September 1995
Second Printing - April 1996

Canadian Cataloguing in Publication Data
Kaufmann, Klaus 1942 -
Kombucha Rediscovered!

Includes bibliographical references and index.
ISBN 0-920470-64-5

1. Tea fungus - Therapeutic use. I. Title.
RM666. T25K38 1995 615' .3292'225 C95-910814-9

Printed and bound in Canada

Dedicated to my devoted mother
who brewed the tastiest tea in the world

Contents

Foreword

Hardly a day goes by, at the Wild Rose College or Clinic, that someone doesn't phone to ask a question about Kombucha tea, "that mushroom tea", or maybe the pancake mushroom tea. The timing couldn't be more appropriate for an informational book on this medicinal substance. Is this just a fad? Popularity has come and gone for this "mushroom tea" over the centuries. Knowledge of it goes back at least 2,000 years. If time is any indication, it is not just a fad. Is it "food from the Gods?" Is it a panacea? Can it cure diseases as diverse as arthritis, baldness and cancer? Those are some of the questions I hope you will have answered in this book.

Kombucha tea can be found in some health shops, but is most often grown at home, handed from friend to friend. This aspect is probably one of the most important issues related to the tea. As Kombucha tea involves a microorganism, careful handling is a must. Many practitioners have suggested it not be used by immuno-compromised people or, because of the sugar levels, by diabetics. Others feel that it should not be used by people who have yeast infections. All of these claims may be true of certain strains and not true of others as all Kombucha teas are not the same basic colony.

I don't believe that any medicinal substance can in itself cure anything, but they can help us on the way to a better quality of life. The use of microorganisms as medicinal substances is not new. Many of the mainstream antibiotics were derived from microorganisms. As well, some people introduce friendly bacteria, such as *acidophilus*, into their diet in the form of yogurt or in capsulated form. Having a proper ecological balance of microorganisms can be quite important to one's state of health. I think we will be hearing many more reports of healing agents coming from the fungal, yeast and bacterial realms. As time goes on, the myths about this tea will either be proven true or false as explanations for its functional reactions with human physiology come forward. If you want to become a Kombucha tea drinker or are curious about what it is, this book is a good place to start.

Terry Willard PhD
Wild Rose College of Natural Healing
September 1995

Publisher's Preface

A modern age dawned and with it came the nightmare of modern food preparation. Refrigeration, pasteurization, canning, processing and freezing may be convenient in our fast-paced society, but they have made our food base devoid of nutrition. They rob food of its vitamins, minerals, enzymes and essential fatty acids. As a result, our century has seen a rise in such frightening diseases as cancer, and people are plagued with chronic diseases of the bowel, stomach and liver. Poor nutrition and thus poor health has led people to search for alternate forms of food and methods of food preparation. Often, people simply rediscover ancient practices.

Lately, there has been a rediscovery of the benefits of lactic acid fermented foods. Lactic acid fermentation is the oldest known method for the preservation of food. To keep vegetables for the winter, our ancestors fermented them and placed them in storage areas built underground that, unlike our modern basements, were not sealed from moisture and air. Many staples in our ancestors' diets were foods preserved in this manner. Whole, raw, unrefined foods and fermented foods such as sourdough bread, kefir, cured meats and natural cheeses, complemented with fresh or fermented fruits and vegetables, provided a nutritional foundation for an active life. Our post-industrial nutritional beliefs tell us that this form of food preparation is primitive and tedious. Yet, a knowledge base so shared and ancient cannot be dismissed so easily. Luckily for us, fermented foods are coming back into fashion.

One might wonder what the benefits of fermented foods would be. It is simple. The fermentation process has been proven to produce a variety of substances from acetylcholine, which benefits the body's nervous system, to choline, which normalizes blood pressure and prevents hypertension. In addition, fermented foods are rich in vitamin C and B and are full of enzymes. Unlike other methods of preserving foods, lactic acid fermentation maintains the life and thus the nutritional value of the microorganism it utilizes. Lactic acids in such foods as yogurt and sauerkraut benefit the human body in more ways than previously imagined. L(+) lactic acid, a direct product of the fermentation process, successfully battles digestive problems by aiding in the expulsion and elimination of unfriendly bacteria and cleansing the bowels. Detoxification is a key principle of optimal health as the elimination of unnecessary substances provides the body with boundless energy and life.

The lost art of proper food preparation was bound to be rediscovered. Most discoveries start with a mystery where only hints and clues are revealed. Kombucha tea, a fermented beverage, is one of those clues. With Kombucha tea added to a balanced diet, the mystery of obtaining ideal health via properly prepared foods is well on the way to being solved.

Acknowledgements

The search for perfect health and the love of writing has guided me throughout my life. Along the way, I have met some great people and have had several striking experiences. They have filled me with the thirst for knowledge. This thirst led to my discovery of Kombucha tea.

I want to offer my very special thanks to my Kombucha gurus, Waltraut Schaffer, Wal Kneifel, Murray Mitchell, Alex Lauder, Sandra Poulton and Dr. Kuni Fann. They have all contributed meaningfully toward "brewing" this mushroom book.

The credit for the idea of this book goes to Kombucha lover and my publisher, Siegfried Gursche. If it were not for the dedicated and professional editing of Gisela Temmel and Katherine Zia, this book would not be so "readable." I thank Ron Crompton, Peter Virag and Lisa Trommeshauser for giving visual appeal to this volume. As always heaps of gratitude to my wife Gabryelle, who is interested in what I am up to and diligently supports my efforts. Finally, special thanks to our beautiful dog Bing, who made sure I would not get lonely by simply curling up at my feet and staying with me for hours on end.

I suppose I ought to eat or drink something or other; but the great question is "What?" There was a large mushroom growing near her, about the same height as herself; and, when she had looked under it, and on both sides of it, and behind it, it occurred to her that she might as well look and see what was on the top of it.

LEWIS CARROLL

We are talking about a "Panacea" Manchurian Mushroom that takes seven days to reproduce itself, it looks like a grayish colored hot cake. It is very fast growing and turns the tea into radical proteins, enzymes and vitamins that work to clean and detoxify your blood very quickly. Properly cultivated it is good for:

1. Eliminates wrinkles and helps removal of brown spots on hands, It's a skin humectant
2. Prevents certain types of cancer in Manchuria, where this mushroom is from, not one case of cancer has been detected. Each day the people drink this tea as a religious atonement.
3. During menopause, reduces hot-flash discomforts. Just after drinking the tea you may feel a warm sensation, due to the fact that the teas components join the blood stream causing a draining action of toxic chemical elements and fluids, the reason for which you will notice increased mobility in your extremities and flexibility around your waist.
4. Helps with constipation.
5. Helps muscular aches and pains in the shoulders and neck.
6. Helps bronchitis, asthma, coughs in 2 days, Helps children with phlegm.
7. Helps with allergies, also with aching nerves.
8. It is prescribed in kidney problems.
9. It's proven useful in cataracts and other formations on the cornea.
10. It cleanses the gall bladder, helps colitis and nervous stomachs.
11. It helps heal diseases. It will lower cholesterol & softens veins & arteries.
12. It will stop infectious diarrhea.
13. Helps burning of fat, therefore it also helps one to lose weight.
14. Helps with insomnia.
15. Helps the liver work more efficiently.
16. Helps to level off glucose, and sudden drops of blood sugar in diabetes. Taken daily, it eliminates urea in 100 days.
17. It has surprising effects on the scalp, it helps avoid balding, thickens hair, helps to eliminate gray hair.
18. Helps digestion.

The Manchurian Mushroom has all of these miraculous properties. It was brought into Mexico from Shogegachum. Manchuria, on the Siberian border.

HOW TO PREPARE YOUR TEA AND PROPAGATE THE MUSHROOM

You must use a glass or enameled pot or container (3 1/2 quart glass pot by Visions is ideal) there can be no metal rim. When you handle the mushroom, take off all of your rings and any other metal that could come into near proximity to the mushroom. If you use a spoon be sure it is wooden plastic or ceramic.

Heat 3 quarts of water, when it starts to boil add I cup of

SPRING WateR OR Distilled ✗ 1-CUP 5 TEA BAG LET STEEP

The role of the infinitely small in nature
is infinitely great.

LOUIS PASTEUR

Introduction

In the late Eighties I saw many sick and overweight people during my travels through the USA and Canada. On my return, I felt moved to write a book on juice fasting for cleansing, slimming and health restoration. In searching out references, I found valuable information, yet somehow did not come across the cleansing value of Kombucha tea. Fasting and cleansing are important contributors to health and well-being. Drinking plenty of nutritional beverages is equally important to overall health. On discovering Kombucha, I developed a positive feeling about the innate restorative value of the Kombucha drink for fasting and detoxifying.

In the early Nineties, I researched and wrote on silica. Soon, I noticed that though in our day and age we may scorn simple remedies, inspired healers as far back in time as the ancient Chinese and Greeks used them constantly and successfully. These mystical medicine men and women of old had deep knowledge of all the natural and simple healing arts. Science is only now slowly rediscovering some of them. Similarly, modern society had forgotten and had to "discover" and promote Kombucha.

This forgetfulness was involved when I was first introduced to the Kombucha mushroom tea. A friendly German woman told me that she had seen a wondrous mushroom years ago on her mother's kitchen shelf in her apartment in downtown Munich. I probed more, but she said she forgot to ask her mother about the mushroom floating in a liquid. Somehow, her mother also forgot to tell her what it was. Years later, in Canada, an acquaintance gave this friend of mine a mushroom, telling her it was a great cure-all. The lady, my friend forgot her name, called it the "Manchurian Mushroom." She gave my friend a hand-me-down leaflet on how to cultivate the "Manchurian." When passed to me, I found the fragmentary instructions so powerful that I have reproduced them here.

(Someone had added the handwritten notes at the bottom and the whole thing was typed on an old typewriter, complete with spelling errors and obvious omissions. To retain the charm and authenticity, the reproduction contains all the original errors.)

Was this perhaps the Kombucha mushroom I wanted to get? The German lady friend told me that she kept it in her fridge and had not reproduced it. She also confirmed that she had never heard of the word "Kombucha" by asking me, "What is it?" She did not know if her mushroom could be the Kombucha mushroom. She had stopped drinking the tea because it did not reproduce in the fridge. Remarkably, she did tell me that a biochemist at the University of British Columbia in Vancouver, BC, Canada had analyzed this Manchurian Mushroom some time ago for the lady who gave it to her. The biochemist had confirmed to her lady friend that the Manchurian was biologically active and did contain a lot of healthy components - just as asserted. I contacted UBC, but unfortunately, could not find the biochemist in question. It seemed that I was on the right track though because the incoming news reports kept mushrooming.

It did not take long to figure out that here indeed, I had a true Kombucha mushroom only known by another name. The Manchurian was not new. "There is nothing new under the sky", the Bible says. Yet, we are prone to forget. Humanity easily forgets because catastrophic events can occur that cause the whole world to forget. When momentary survival is at stake, ancient health secrets are forgotten overnight.

Such were the enmity and hatred between the advanced nations in the first half of the Twentieth Century that two world wars resulted. People all over the world forgot not only the most important aspects of life such as peace and tranquillity, but also the healing abilities of certain foods and drinks. In the aftermath of two world wars and heavy regional wars after that (Korea, Vietnam, Afghanistan), people were busy fighting or marching for peace. Only today, in the new age of relative peace and security, do we enjoy the leisure to look after our physical and spiritual health. Due to increasing longevity, there is even a dire necessity to stay well. Governments can no longer afford to pay for health care.

People are searching for alternate ways to cope with health complaints. Thus, remedies like Kombucha tea are coming back to us just in time.

Writing some years ago on treatment modes for cancer, I noticed that reevaluating a generally known natural treatment, a food or drink like sauerkraut or lactic acid fermented juices, is extremely important. Not only for those who are suffering from a cancer, but also for those who are delivering health care (in the better sense of that word) to ourselves, to our family, our friends and neighbors - in short, to all of us. The value of a lactic acid fermented drink, I soon discovered, is intimately connected to Kombucha tea.

So I think of this work merely as a revival of ancient knowledge. There is evidence as we will find out, that the ancients created Kombucha. They knew more of the friendly and beneficial coexistence of different life forms than today's researchers of symbiosis. Much like Alice in Wonderland, humanity got lost on its way through the timeless eons. Much like Alice, from time to time we all need someone to remind us of the good things in life. From Wonderland, we all know of the mushroom that Alice eats on the advice of the caterpillar. Well then, this Kombucha book takes on, as will become apparent, the role of the direction-giving caterpillar, though I advise against smoking the pipe.

"One side will make you grow taller, and
the other side will make you grow shorter."
"One side of what? The other side of what?"
thought Alice to herself.
"Of the mushroom," said the Caterpillar.
ALICE IN WONDERLAND

Part 1

WHAT A FUNNY LOOKIN' FUNGUS!

The foods that prolong life and increase purity, vigour, health, cheerfulness, and happiness are those that are delicious, soothing, substantial and agreeable.

Bhagavad Gita (c. 400 BC)

Chapter One

What's It All About?

Much More Energy

I shut my eyes as I guzzled down the first draught. I had briefly tasted a tiny bit of the ciderlike tea that came with my first Kombucha mushroom and so I was totally unprepared for this taste treat. My first Kombucha drink tasted like French bubbly despite the negligible alcohol content. I will never forget this great taste experience. I was thrilled like I had not been in years.

Imagine your favorite drink being suddenly simultaneously energizing and superhealthy, and you have Kombucha in a nutshell. Its fizziness and sweetness are two reasons why people enjoy drinking Kombucha tea. This fabulous tea ranges in taste from sweet champagne (right after harvest), to wine, beer, apple cider and even cola. Also, it is without the detriment to well-being that the commercial alcoholic and carbonated beverages have. Knowing the general public's preferences for sweetness, fizz and pop, clever manufacturers incorporate the pleasant tongue tingling by carbonizing their commercial drinks. They have found this to improve sales. Then, they add gallons of sugar. Most people love and cannot live without sugar. By that hangs a sugary tale that we will explore anon.

If you, like me, enjoy a healthy, thirst quenching drink that tastes and bubbles like champagne when fresh, and tastes and smells like refreshing cider when refrigerated, come on board. Read on. If you had given up hope of finding a magic potion that can energize, rejuvenate and taste good, you can now come alive with a new "miracle mushroom" tea that will quench your thirst and reenergize you.

You will not miss the taste of champagne, beer, cider, or cola. It is a promise. Kombucha will keep you happy all around. Come again . . . Komb . . . what? Kombucha. Some readers may know of Kombucha, but I will explain what Kombucha means and what it is all about for those who have not heard of it.

If nature ever bestowed the amazing grace of combining health benefits with a refreshing taste, Kombucha is it. No need for the upset stomach you get after too much cola or champagne. Kombucha is so good, the second thing you will notice is how it soothes your stomach. (First you will notice the taste.) Kombucha gives you new vitality within minutes of drinking. So what is this panacea?

Simply speaking, Kombucha is a tea. It looks like tea. It smells like tea. I am a tea expert, so to speak. My mother weaned me on tea. I learned the pleasure and the art of the tea ceremony from her. My mother made the best tasting tea in the world, whether green, black or herbal. If she had known about Kombucha she might not have died at such a young age. However, in postwar Germany the people had forgotten about the health benefits of Kombucha tea.

I first heard about Kombucha tea from Waltraut Schaffer, who brought it from Germany and made it for herself to treat her digestive troubles. According to Waltraut, her digestion promptly improved upon drinking Kombucha. She was just a little concerned about the sugar in Kombucha. As we will see, there is ultimately no reason to be concerned, because most of the sugar is converted before the tea is ready to drink.

I got my first Kombucha mushroom from Sandra Poulton. I live in Vancouver, British Columbia. Sandra lives in Lions Head in Northern Ontario on the peninsula of land that divides Georgian Bay from Lake Huron. She wrapped my Kombucha "baby" in plastic. She sealed it in a plastic bag, floating it in some of its own juice, and couriered it to me. Two days later, I saw my first Kombucha. Sandra had told me that she started fermenting her first Kombucha culture in the spring of 1995. She got her baby from a friend and has since been successfully brewing Kombucha tea. Sandra, who lets her tea ferment from seven to ten days, compares the taste of the tea to apple cider.

Sandra states, "I however drink Kombucha mainly not for its thirst quenching ability but for its health bestowing properties.

I quite like it. The taste is very similar to apple cider. It's quite pleasant to drink. On average I let it ripen for seven to ten days. It's usually ready at that point. You can tell because it will become very fragrant. When the weather is hot, I use seven days, so in the heat of summer I can have it off quicker. In winter it is a little cooler, so it takes a little longer." Her friend's Kombucha has since died. So Sandra returned the favor by giving her friend one of her babies, as it were. Sandra keeps her Kombucha warm and covers it with a couple sheets of newspaper during the fermentation process. She just throws the newspaper lightly over top of the bowl in which the Kombucha is floating. She does not keep it in absolute darkness.

Sandra says, "I don't know if it is just imagination, but the roots of my grey hairs are taking on new color. I find it a bit early to say for sure because I've only been using the Kombucha for about three months. Because hair grows rather slowly, it is too soon to tell." Then she adds that her friend says that her own Kombucha drinking had started removing the age spots on her hands. "I have a general concern to stay healthy," says Sandra, who has been practicing prevention for some time. She drinks Kombucha mainly to keep up her program of preventive health care. "I don't have any major problems right now, and I don't want any!" Then, she cautions, "the taste might be a bit overwhelming for newcomers to Kombucha because it can be quite sharp. Yet if you can drink apple cider vinegar, you can drink Kombucha."

Bonny Therapy

Having tasted my first Kombucha and been convinced, I was now getting more interested in its apparent health restorative abilities. I discussed Kombucha with acupuncturist, certified herbalist and student of Chinese medicine, Bonnie Mori of B & B Farms in Niagara-on-the-Lake, Ontario. She says, "My experience with Kombucha is now seven months. Before that, I was searching for it for five years! Now, besides drinking it regularly myself, I prescribe Kombucha to my clients for many conditions and invariably, they meet with success. I have also recommended it to my entire family and friends for digestive ailments, for constipation, belching, gas, and lack of energy. Depending on cases, I use Kombucha with live cell therapy and homeopathy. I know of at least one person who, besides drinking it regularly, uses Kombucha as an astringent. This person successfully combatted acne and claims to have less oily hair as well since using Kombucha from within and from outside on the skin and hair."

"How do you and your clients find the taste?" I ask. Bonnie confirms what I already know, "Frankly, it tastes to me like bubbly champagne when it is fresh. That's when I like it best, fresh and still warm. After cooling a bit in the fridge, it becomes like apple cider. It all depends a bit on how long I let it ferment. I usually let it sit for ten days, but not in this heat, it takes less." (Our talk takes place at the end of June 1995. Ontario swelters in a heat wave.)

Bonnie continues, "Some of my clients have told me, I look younger than ever and all of them always confirm, much more energy." One said, "I had just a glass in the morning. Couldn't believe it but I was up till 12:30 at night and feeling fine." Another says, "No more coffee for me. Now my wife uses it to clear up her constipation." At this point in our conversation, Bonnie grows more animated and confides, "Some people got instantaneously more energy for the rest of the day after drinking Kombucha. I gave it, for instance, to a top manager at GM who is living in my area. He likes to play hockey as a counterbalance to his sedentary occupation. His game had slackened off. Now he has energy for two games. I have even given it to one diabetic to fight off her diarrhea. It worked and she even obtained some desired weight loss."

"Great, but what about all the sugar in the Kombucha?" I ask. "Oh, she ferments it for fourteen days and after that there's no sugar left. It has all been converted," Bonnie replies and continues, "I think Kombucha acts as a catalyst in the body and thus causes all kinds of beneficial changes. That part of it may not work as rapidly. I think the quick energizing that people notice almost immediately is due to the amino acids and the vitamins in the tea fungus. That is what users instantaneously absorb."

Then Bonnie tells me of another case she treated, "This fellow burped all night and could not sleep a wink. Since drinking the Kombucha tea, the burping has stopped and he sleeps like a baby." Bonnie adds, "I even give the tea to my cats and dogs. I find that they are less prone to infections that they used to contract especially around here at this time of year." At the end of our conversation I ask, "Any final words on Kombucha for my readers?" After a bit of reflection Bonnie says, "Well, it sounds really weird, but it's like this. Most of my clients say, 'I cannot believe that I'm taking this home.' They are so afraid of the opinion of others, or that they may look ridiculous in someone else's eyes. So they find it sometimes a bit difficult to adopt a Kombucha baby, but once they are drinking the tea and feeling the difference, they continue and by and by pass along the tea and the gospel to their family, friends, and neighbors."

Free Kombucha Homeopathy

Alex Lauder of Guelph, Ontario is a homeopathic practitioner who employs the Kombucha mushroom tea in his daily practice. Lauder recommends Kombucha to his patients mainly as an adjunct to a multidisciplinary homeopathic program for cancer patients. During our conversation, Lauder tells me that, "as part of the program and whenever patients need antioxidants, I suggest Kombucha. I know of cases where remission occurred that could only be ascribed to the Kombucha. We have seen lumps disappear from under the skin of Kombucha users."

Lauder emphasizes that he provides the Kombucha free of charge to his patients and that there is no profit motive involved in his Kombucha treatment. Better perhaps than any scientific studies is the fact that Kombucha tea is a healing agent available either at a low cost or free. The undeniable fact that no one is making a fortune off Kombucha underlines its obvious success and usefulness as a remedy. Lauder then tells me that though he has not witnessed any spontaneous energizing of people who drink the tea, his wife has been using it for some time on her face as well as drinking it regularly. He can confirm that her skin looks younger than ever and that her facial lines have disappeared. Meanwhile, his mother at the healthy age of eighty-two, is benefiting from Kombucha tea.

When I ask him if he ever finds that his patients experience difficulties keeping the mushroom alive and reproducing, he smiles, "only the purists who insist on using brown sugar instead of white." Then he confirms that most people do not have difficulties 'giving birth' to healthy Kombucha babies and raising them. After ending my conversation with Mr. Lauder, I felt even more encouraged because Kombucha tea and therapy have obviously found acceptance in some practitioners in the respected medical discipline of Homeopathy.

Recapturing the Active Life

At a recent Kombucha lecture given by Betsy Pryor in Las Vegas, Nevada during the annual NNFA (National Nutritional Foods Association) convention, they asked what participants gained from drinking Kombucha. These typical answers show how people benefited: "My complexion is cleared up and I've lost weight. Minimal, but I feel I just want to eat less." "I drank it for quite a while and I noticed I had better digestion and I really feel it has helped my liver. My son uses it when it's hot weather and he is in construction and does cement work. And he says he can drink a full glass of this on the job and has his thirst quenched or he can drink a gallon of water and feel terrible afterwards and it doesn't help."

Others reported, "It helps me with my menopause. It just balances me through the hot flashes. I'm just sliding through it." "It's really helped my skin. I always had like teenage breakouts. I don't have those anymore. Besides that, my son, I've had my son on it now about four months. He's twenty-six years old and almost bald. He says, 'Mom, I'm getting hair. My hair is coming back.'" "I started taking it just a few weeks ago. My first immediate notice was just more energy, and you feel like you get a great night of sleep. I sleep less but feel like, wow, I slept great."

Between these testimonials, Betsy Pryor relates how at age forty-nine she lost fourteen pounds after drinking Kombucha tea for two months. Though she does not work out much, her muscles became harder. Then, after one year of drinking Kombucha, she noticed her grey hairs were disappearing. Now that she has been drinking it for two years, her hair has thickened and has never been as long. Also, she reports sleeping less but being more focused. She even noticed that she is developing a photographic memory. Then, she tells the audience that Kombucha has become the drink of choice for many Hollywood actors, who use it instead of artificial stimulants to get them through their sixteen hour days.

According to writer and researcher Harald W. Tietze, the Russian military regularly drinks Kombucha. He also reports that Kombucha underwent trials in the German military, the "Bundeswehr." The Army Sports School in Germany under Professor Dr. Simon Gerrit reportedly concluded that, "pure biological Kombucha fermented tea" has a "strengthening effect and improves the performances of the athletes." The German soldiers reportedly drank 200 ml of Kombucha three times a day. Their average training times improved. The muscles of a hardworking soldier's body give off more lactic acid with the break down of glycogen. We know this process as glycolysis. The German army doctors concluded that Kombucha appreciably reduces glycolysis.

Also athletes reportedly recovered quicker from their exertions. Tests done by Dr. Wiesner confirmed these findings. More tests reconfirmed them at the Olympic training ground in Warendorf in Münsterland, Germany. There, they tested twelve trained athletes by running various parameters first without and then with 200 ml per day of Kombucha tea.

Blood samples were taken throughout the various tests. The results confirmed that the athletes achieved better training times with the Kombucha tea. The team of physicians in charge noticed in particular the markedly lowered lactate values in the blood (i.e. the salts of lactic acid). In addition, reportedly all participating athletes felt more energetic and recovered quickly after the runs involving Kombucha therapy. The scientists concluded that Kombucha led to positive changes in the energy metabolism of the cells. An ability to affect cellular energy exchanges could explain the increase in physical ability and the increased well-being the athletes experienced.

Not surprisingly, in Russia, trainers give high performance athletes Kombucha tea to increase energy output. There have even been reports in the European health magazines about Kombucha being given to racing camels in Arab countries although the total composition of the camel 'dope' was kept a proprietary secret.

A Healthy Thirst Quencher for Children

Not just soldiers and athletes benefit, ordinary people of all ages from all over the globe reap the rewards of drinking Kombucha tea. In their book *Kombucha Phenomenon*, writers Betsy Pryor and Sanford Holst literally flood readers with impressive testimonials from Kombucha drinkers from different occupations and regions of the US, including some of the rich and famous across their great country.

The most famous Kombucha researcher, Rosina Fasching, recommends Kombucha tea even for children. However, she points out that the drink usually contains a bit of theine, a form of caffeine contained in black tea, which could stimulate children. Apart from that, if yogurt is good for children, Kombucha should be even better. It offers the additional advantage of not posing a problem for children that have a lactose intolerance and may be unable to digest milk products properly. All the references I found recommend the drink for children. To make it more palatable for children, it can be easily diluted with their favorite fruit juice, or simply with water.

Protection against Cancer

If you need more reasons for this thirst quencher, how about this. In a recent article in Canada's *Financial Post* (fp-Review-Health, July 15, 1995), Dr. W. Gifford-Jones reports, "Dr. Wei Zheng, assistant professor of epidemiology at the University of Minnesota, has good news for tea drinkers. Researchers studied 42,000 women between the ages of fifty-five and sixty-nine for seven years. Daily tea drinkers showed a 75% decrease in risk of cancer in the upper-digestive organs and a 60% reduction in the risk of kidney cancer compared with non-tea drinkers." The report goes on to confirm that "Zheng does not know the nature of this protective mechanism. But green and black tea contain polyphenols, which are strong antioxidants like vitamins C and E." Adding all we have seen so far together, it seems certain that with the help of regular drinking of Kombucha tea, we can effectively prolong our longevity.

Reaching 100 with Kombucha

Are you ready for "from the cradle to immortality?" You and I may be, but most people are afraid of longevity. They associate old age with negative feelings about infirmity, poverty and loneliness. Yet none of this need be so. Perhaps the best is yet to come? This reminds me of the poetic line "do not go gentle into that good night. Rage, rage against the dying of the light." (Dylan Thomas, 1946)

When we moved into a new home three years ago, I found a stone sculpture of the number 100. I was delighted because it was also the year of my 50th birthday. I took the sculpture to be a positive sign.

Will I reach 100? With Kombucha helping to retain firmness of flesh, energy of muscles and sinews and a keen enjoyment of living, why not indeed? I can directly connect one name for Kombucha to increased longevity. In Russia, Kombucha became famous as "Kargasok tea" because the Kargasok region in Russia is renowned for the longevity of its people. They reportedly drink copious amounts of the tea throughout their long lives.

Could all these benefits be true? Half of what happens to us happens because we believe it to be true. Psychology calls this phenomenon the power of the mind. The Bible calls it a miracle. Science calls it the placebo effect. I suspect they are all right. If you want something badly enough, you will attain it. Perhaps the word "will" is instrumental here. In any event, some centenarians ascribe their longevity to Kombucha drinking. It might be true. Personally, I will not argue with it, but will put it to the test. I am writing this book in 1995. I will be turning 100 in 2042. You will be hearing from me. You will probably catch me sipping Kombucha tea, but not in a wheelchair or in a bed. I will be busy gardening, travelling and writing my memoirs. I will have many miracles to tell. One thing is for sure, I am inspired by my 100 sign and aided by my Kombucha tea.

Are you seeking the Greatest? Let the plant instruct you.
What it is without will, willingly be it - that's it!
SCHILLER

Chapter Two

A Refreshing Tea

Major Uses and Health Benefits

We should not expect too many healing and preventive properties from what is primarily an excellent health drink with a superb taste, possibly exceeding that of beer and wine for a fraction of the cost. Kombucha tea is or should be drunk mainly for its excellent taste. In any event, it is superior for health than either alcoholic bubblies such as champagne, cider or beer, or stomach upsetting carbonated soft drinks.

Yet medical history has recorded many therapeutic benefits for Kombucha tea. Especially in Russia, where the tea has a lively history, the people often observed healing effects occurring after regularly drinking their Kombucha kvass. The healing benefits are varied, so there has been a tendency to recommend Kombucha for all disease states. That, of course, leads to suggestions of dishonesty. No wonder that some writers shy away from making medicinal claims. Nevertheless, since few people profit from selling the tea, I have trouble with the dishonesty criticism.

Benefits from drinking the Kombucha beverage are most likely due to its cleansing, detoxifying and acidifying effects, and the polyphenols or weak acids with antioxidant properties. Many Kombucha experts recommend the Kombucha tea as a diuretic in edemas, in arteriosclerosis, in cases of gout, sluggish bowels, for stones and as a refreshment or, after longer fermenting, a food vinegar. The experts praise the tea for its toning of the entire metabolism and its normalizing effect on cell membranes, which increases overall well-being. Experience has also shown the tea to regulate the intestinal flora, to strengthen the cells, to harmonize the metabolism, to function as a natural antibiotic, and to help maintain the pH, the acid-alkaline balance of the body. Finally, according to testimonials and expert findings, Kombucha strengthens the immune response.

There are also reports about Kombucha's usefulness when applied directly to the skin. Apart from its rejuvenating qualities on the skin of the face, as reported to me by a homeopathic doctor, Kombucha tea application from within and without can help to retain or restore beautiful, wrinkle-free skin. This is apparently a boon that Kombucha shares with silica gel. I believe that any thorough skin care program using Kombucha tea should be incorporating silica gel. Kombucha experts have recommended beauty baths with Kombucha tea. Despite some arguments to the contrary (that hold that the skin hermetically seals us from outside influences), I agree with experts who maintain that the skin can absorb healing substances like silica and Kombucha from without.

These experts include Maria Treben, Rudolf Breuss and the world's foremost herbal medicine expert, Rudolf Fritz Weiss. We can best treat skin and connective tissue problems from within and without simultaneously. Come to think of it, what could be more relaxing than enjoying a cleansing bath while simultaneously causing gentle healing. Of course, Kombucha tea also lends itself to compresses and poultices when beneficial for skin conditions. Trauma to skin (wounds, ulcers etc.), muscle tissue, skin eruptions, rheumatic pains and fevers all respond well to external applications of Kombucha tea.

The Longer I Use Kombucha the Better I Feel

I have heard from regular users of Kombucha tea that their keen enjoyment of living increases the longer they use Kombucha tea. Many find they can do things again for which they previously did not have the energy. Arguing with this is hard, but I hold we should not use any supplement or remedy continuously or over long periods without an occasional break. There is evidence that the effect of any remedy or panacea diminishes if continued without a natural break in the pattern. Good healers therefore recommend adopting a regimen that has an on/off pattern. It does not matter how you organize this, as long as it is done.

For instance, a regimen of five days on, two days off, would work for some. A regimen of five weeks on, two weeks off or five months on, two months off would suit others. Take your pick depending on your needs and lifestyle. This pattern is not only more in tune with the natural rhythm of life, but also less costly to users of health supplements. Then, when we are under special stress or become gravely ill, we can continue the usage of healing agents for a longer period until we feel well again and are ready for another break in the pattern.

Slim and Feeling Great Thanks to Kombucha

Most experts also agree that feeling great and being slim go hand in hand. Despite the stereotyped jollity of many an overweight person, their condition, which makes them prone to blood pressure problems, usually also makes them wish it were not so. They wish so, strangely enough, not only for health considerations, but also for considerations of the personal ego and increasing perceived appeal for improved physical appearance. Given the facts, we should all be perfectly poised and balanced individuals. Yet this is not true. So what exactly is it that keeps a slim person slim and an overweight person overweight?

Apart from dietary considerations, the incredible force of habit plus a possible problem with the setting of the internal appestat (the biological switch for controlling appetite messages from brain and stomach), metabolic disorders play a large role in being overweight. Anything that can exercise an influence on these four points, ego appeal, diet, appetite, and the metabolism, will be of great help. The first thing that comes to mind is, of course, exercise. As the saying goes, "no pain, no gain." All medical experts agree that exercise will keep us slim and feeling great. Kombucha can help to make this come true for us by energizing us into action through metabolic healing, thus making the exercise activity far more enjoyable.

Is Kombucha tea fattening? The caloric values of Kombucha are difficult to establish with any accuracy. However, according to Günther W. Frank, who had some fun calculating the calories in the tea, the argument goes as follows: White sugar has 394 kilo calories (kcal). If seventy grams per liter are used for the fermentation process of the tea, it produces 276 kcal. Of course, the fermentation process uses up a great portion of the sugar. Given a residual sugar content of 30g per liter, Frank arrives at 118 kcal. On lowering this to 20g per liter the result becomes 79 kcal. Also, the longer the tea is fermenting, ten days rather than seven, the lower the residual sugar content. That is that folks. Keep in mind that the sugar is in the tea for one reason only, to feed the mushroom.

Taking in daily about 2,500 kilo calories is generally sufficient nourishment for people who do light work, like office work. It would not be enough for industrial workers or constructions workers and is not recommended for the sick without approval from their health practitioner. If you are embarking on a slimming adventure and want to boost your digestive tract for quicker elimination, now is the time to start drinking a glass of Kombucha tea ten minutes after every meal. That way you can lose weight without fasting.

Adding The Joy of Juice Fasting

Famous people like Elizabeth Taylor and Oprah Winfrey spent millions of dollars a year at "fat farms" to obtain weight loss the expensive way. (Liz Taylor paid money to have to sweep the kitchen at the Betty Ford Clinic!) Yet anyone can fast easily and pleasantly with the aid of Kombucha and other fermented liquids. In my book, *The Joy of Juice Fasting*, I explain the beauty and rewards of fasting and the special advantages of lactic acid fermented juices that aid fasting. I recommend this book to users of the Kombucha tea who want to undertake a guided day-by-day cleansing fast using the Kombucha tea.

Living organisms can be (successfully)
combatted by live matter only!
ENDERLEIN

Chapter Three

The Revitalizing Life in the Tea

Unseen Friends for Life

Raising a Kombucha is like taking a minicourse in microbiology because the Kombucha mushroom is a conglomeration of microorganisms. Since the Kombucha beverage is a collaboration of certain bacteria and certain yeast cultures, with ourselves as transient host and beneficiaries, why not become friends for life with the Kombucha culture.

Humankind has made beer for years and uses a living culture for this brewing process. So it is with wine and most alcohols. Since time immemorial, we also make yogurt, cheeses, kefir and sourdough breads with living yeast and bacterial cultures. Many of our best foods (cultured butter is superior to other butter) stem from living cultures as well. Live food is essential to the well-being of any creature. Without friendly microbes, humans and all other life forms could not survive for long. In turn, all fungi and most bacteria depend on other living organisms for food.

Beneficial Symbiosis

The microbes in Kombucha are not pathogens out to harm us. Instead they live together for mutual benefit. The most compelling example of what is beneficial symbiosis involves termites. These insects are very aggravating to people who live in wooden houses because the termites eat wood. They eat it, but they cannot digest the cellulose of which the living tree makes the wood fibers. So how does it get digested? Inside every termite's intestines live tiny protozoans with the capacity for digesting wood. When somehow deprived of these protozoans, a termite literally starves to death, no matter how much wood it may consume. Another beneficial symbiosis is known as lichen, which is, in reality, a close association of algae and fungi.

Humanity has long ago discovered the benefits of using symbioses in important food and drink preparations. In wine making, the grape juice (called Must) is processed primarily by a yeast called *Saccharomyces cerevisiae var. ellipsoideus*. Cider and Japanese saki are other examples of culture ferments. As we know, the fermenting results in pleasant drinks, which are popular the world over. The fermented Kombucha beverage is equally tasty, but much less expensive (costing no more than a regular cup of tea), easy to make and a worthwhile remedy if made and used correctly. Remember that even coffee and chocolate owe their final flavor to beneficial microbial activity.

We rarely stop to think about it, but many of our most important friends (and enemies - we'll get into that one later), are usually invisible to us because they are too small to make out with the unaided eye. We call the field of science that treats of invisible life forms microbiology. We call the permanent or long lasting association of microbes, symbiosis (living together for mutual benefit). Symbiosis is a widespread phenomenon. The world of the living is a web of interrelated life forms.

Many such symbiotic relationships exist on and in human beings which serve and protect us while helping some of our metabolic actions that could not take place otherwise. Kombucha is a particularly healthy symbiosis for the human body and not one that is either automatic or permanent. The Kombucha components, it would appear, are beneficial transients in our bodies. We could compare them with a visit from a rich uncle who leaves us in better shape by bestowing on us some of his wealth before departing again. We would want to invite him over repeatedly and then some more.

Due to the fact that it is a living process, depending on regional differences for its survival, the Kombucha symbioses will always be different from place to place. I know that we are dreadfully afraid of bacterial infection, and rightly so. However, there are many friendly bacteria such as *lactobacilli* or *bifidobacteria*, which when added to our regular diet create only beneficial and long lasting healthy effects. Most people consume and enjoy yogurt without even thinking that they are consuming live bacteria.

According to research done in Moscow, the symbiotic partners consist of Bacterium *zylinum* and yeast cells of the genus *Saccharomyces*. Other friendly symbiotes possibly present are according to researcher Frank, *Saccharomyces ludwigii*, *Saccharomyces apiculatus*, Bacterium *xylinoides*, Bacterium *gluconicum*, *Schizo saccharomyces pombe*, *Acetobacter ketogenum*, *Torula* types, *Pichia* fermentans and other yeasts. The yeast cells are the ones that eat the sugar and by consuming it, change it to ethyl alcohol (ethanol) and carbon dioxide.

Meanwhile, the bacteria change the sugar into cellulose. This process enables the mushroom floating on top of the sweetened tea to grow. Yet that is not all. The bacteria ferment the alcohol manufactured by the yeast cells into acetic acid and other organic acids. This means that the Kombucha tea is increasingly soured. Now, disease causing germs cannot reside in the Kombucha tea because only the yeast can withstand the alcohol, which acts as a poison for germs. The fermenting yeast is however acid-proof. In other words, the bacteria protect the yeast who in turn deliver the food on which the bacteria can grow. The two symbiotic partners profit from each other. On their own, neither could continue to exist for long, nor produce the health benefits for the human being who drinks Kombucha tea.

How True Are the Health Benefits?

Not one scientific study (*in vitro* and *in vivo*) exists to confirm the health benefits of the Kombucha symbiosis. We can only say that the benefits are as true as the many personal testimonials and there are a lot. We must bear in mind that remedies don't work for everyone, nor can they work if the body is exposed to deadly toxins.

Some years back a TV documentary showed a female cancer patient slowly dying of her disease over a period of some years. This patient never showed any signs of recovery despite all kinds of treatments. Strangely enough, as I pointed out repeatedly even as I watched the program aghast, this woman smoked cigarettes until the day she died. She had not quit smoking for the sake of her health. She died, probably from smoking.

The Kombucha symbiotes do not tolerate tobacco smoke. Exposed to tobacco smoke during fermentation, the mushroom will not prosper and may die. Be on the lookout for deadly toxins when brewing Kombucha tea to heal your health complaints. Tobacco, we should remind ourselves, is such a deadly poison that farmers are successfully employing it as an insecticide.

Before looking closer at the health benefits of Kombucha tea, we must realize that Kombucha is not a miracle potion. Others such as Christopher Hobbs, have warned against expecting a miracle. They have pointed to the disappointing experiences of many people with substances such as Essiac, Pau d'Arco and Taheebo. Unlike stated in the anonymous instructions for the Manchurian Mushroom reprinted in the introduction, Kombucha is not a panacea for mortality. No one can continuously endanger his or her health and think they can get away with it by sipping a little Kombucha tea once or twice a day. How many people have said, "I just don't know. I was always very healthy, but then, I had a heart attack."

Germans, are very fond of quoting this proverb, "The jug continues going to the fountain until it breaks." If we take good care of our jug, our body, it will last a long time. If, on the other hand, we abuse it, it will break prematurely. Efficacy reports are sometimes contradictory. Let us now look at the main health effects of Kombucha tea. The following is an overview on how we can use Kombucha for various conditions, to help prevent the onset of illness and to help us stay healthy well into old age.

AIDS (Acquired Immune Deficiency Syndrome):

Stories about helping AIDS abound. I had the opportunity to work with AIDS patients, having been involved with Vancouver's AZT trial at St. Paul's Hospital some years ago. This highly publicized ailment is a syndrome rather than a single disease. The impaired immune system needs help. In 1991, we knew that once the disease is active, there isn't a cure. Despite AZT, AIDS victims died within two years of disease manifestation. In 1995, medical science has apparently extended this to three years and new experimental drugs are on the market. Do any work? Who knows? No doubt, caution is advisable before AIDS patients experiment on their own with any homemade remedies promising better T-cell counts. However, according to Kombucha researcher Betsy Pryor, Kombucha tea, while not capable of curing AIDS victims, can help boost immunity and thereby help keep the virus contained for a longer period of time. This possible benefit from the Kombucha culture is presently under study. Seeking the advice of a holistic health practitioner is a good step before employing self-medication.

Arthritis:

This is a complex disease. There are anecdotes from individuals who have reported healing effects from drinking Kombucha tea. Many dancers are drinking Kombucha tea, both in Russia and North America. They are reporting fewer ligament and arthritic problems, something athletes and dancers are prone to suffer. However, natural medicine recommends a comprehensive and holistic therapy for this condition.

Asthma:

Asthma patients under the care of Dr. A. Wiesner noticed considerable improvements while on Kombucha tea therapy.

Blood Pressure (High):

Typically this may be closely connected to high blood lipid or cholesterol levels. This persistent health problem has many causes and many cures. However, regular drinking of Kombucha tea has been known to lower high blood pressure. I would recommend adding silica to the daily diet as well to elasticize the blood vessels.

Bowels:

Kombucha tea can help heal so many illnesses of the stomach and the bowels, that I could write a whole book about it. Kombucha tea shows good results in clearing up stomach and bowel problems by balancing the pH and the intestinal flora. Healing follows automatically once all the body's systems are in good working order.

Bronchitis:

According to Tietze, a Dutch doctor by the name of Harnisch successfully prescribed Kombucha tea for his juvenile patients.

Candida albicans:

This is a type of yeast infection, so it is natural to assume sufferers should stay away from other yeast cultures. Nevertheless, the highly specialized yeast cells in Kombucha help fight off their evil Candida cousins. That, in fact, is the whole secret behind successful symbiosis involving us as hosts. A recent testimonial on Candida I heard in Las Vegas spoke of a fifty year old tax accountant with a yeast infection. She was spending about $30.00 a month on prescription drugs. Three weeks after starting to drink Kombucha, she stopped taking these drugs and has not used them since. Her problems have disappeared. Expert guidance from a naturopath is advisable before beginning Kombucha therapy and to ensure that active yeast cells are living in the tea on harvest day.

Cholesterol:

We all know that high blood lipids (excessive cholesterol) and hypertension (high blood pressure) ultimately lead to heart disease. Since heart disease is still the number one killer in North America, we had better watch our blood lipids. Kombucha tea has been found to lower cholesterol levels.

Chronic Fatigue:

Many researchers report that people told them that Kombucha tea overcame their Chronic Fatigue Syndrome (CFS). If chronic fatigue is due to intestinal and/or liver problems, as some people believe, Kombucha tea, with its cleansing and balancing abilities, could be a key factor in avoiding and overcoming chronic fatigue.

Colds:

Cold viruses take hold of us mainly when we are stressed, tired or depressed, or because a lowered immune response lets us down. Kombucha functions also as a natural antibiotic, so regular Kombucha tea drinking can help prevent or alleviate colds. Adding vitamin C and echinacea to a cold prevention program is vital.

Constipation:

Constipation is often chronic and just as often due to unhealthy foods or insufficient exercise. Much like diarrhea, constipation has reportedly been cleared up quickly by Kombucha tea. Perhaps it is because drinking Kombucha helps to restore the intestinal flora, which in turn overcomes the irritable bowel syndrome. Another habit to prevent constipation is assuring a sufficient daily intake of roughage. Roughage becomes more important with age, because the entire metabolism tends to become a bit sluggish and needs all the encouragement it can get. Roughage, can be a pleasant and enjoyable meal by itself such as green salads, whole grain breads or fruits. With Kombucha tea and regular green salads, you will likely not suffer from constipation. Including roughage and Kombucha in your diet is the best kind of laxative. According to experts and testimonials, even the infamous prune treatment should not be needed after a Kombucha treatment.

Diarrhea:

Kombucha tea seems to clear this problem up quickly. Scientific studies from Russia report that bacterial dysentery responds well to Kombucha.

Fluid Retention:

Testimonials support findings that Kombucha tea can reduce excessive fluid in the legs.

Gout:

One approach to this illness of too much rich food is through the intestines. A balancing of the intestinal flora and a stepped up metabolism, both of which Kombucha tea encourages, could be helpful against gout. Also, juice fasting that incorporates Kombucha tea could alleviate this disease.

Immunity:

If energizing and metabolic activating are the major functions of Kombucha tea, we need say little more as such restorative action will automatically foster the immune system. However, I would suggest that we must also adopt a holistic lifestyle and careful diet with a focus on an ongoing detoxification program to successfully overcome immune impairment. This is particularly true with severe impairment, such as poisoning of the liver or HIV-infection. Other diseases like cancer are similarly bound to be overcome easier with an immune system operating at full capacity. Of course, ultimately, all of us want a functioning immune response. Kombucha tea drinking seems a move in the right direction, although some authors caution against it and advise further research before using Kombucha for HIV or AIDS cases.

Impotence:

It is almost unbelievable how many dollars are being spent searching for a cure for impotency. The German magazine *Der Stern* reported that Germans alone spent 790 million Marks in one year (1992) purchasing sex hormones. Well then, in Kombucha tea we have at long last a panacea for impotence. This is especially so because, unless there is a physical or severe mental disability, potency goes hand in hand with vitality. Dr. Sklenar and others have reported on the toning effect Kombucha tea can have on the male sex organ.

Kidneys:

Among other therapies, adequate amounts of healthy liquids are necessary to flush the kidneys and keep them in top shape. Drinking Kombucha tea could aid healthy kidney flushing. According to Harald W. Tietze, comparison trials conducted by Dr. A. Wiesner resulted in an 89% success rate of Kombucha versus an interferon drug.

MS (Multiple Sclerosis):

Betsy Pryor reports impressive testimonial evidence of MS healing. Also, Harald W. Tietze reports on a Mrs. M. W. from Holland who claimed healing results from Kombucha tea. According to a letter published in the Dutch magazine *Op Zoek* she started drinking Kombucha in April of 1989. Apparently the tea detoxified her entire body. Today she has more energy and even got her driver's license back. Her letter, dated February 1992, states that she plans to go skiing again after taking Kombucha for six months. Obviously there will need to be more clinical studies to confirm this encouraging experience of one individual before giving hope to other MS sufferers.

Prostate:

Prostate problems are common in older men, amounting to some 50% of the over fifty population. The problem can be countered in many ways. Even orthodox medicine is increasingly recognizing that surgery may not be the answer to prostate cancer. Apparently drinking Kombucha tea regularly decreases bladder inflammation and therefore can alleviate prostate inflammation as well. Other prostate remedies include pumpkin seeds, zinc supplements and willow. I suffered severe prostate pain some years ago. Immediately, I embarked on a regular program of supplementing with zinc and willow herb, and eating pumpkin seeds with my cereal. I have not had any prostate pain since adding Kombucha tea therapy to the list of valuable treatment options.

Psoriasis:

Some doctors reportedly recommend Kombucha tea drinking for psoriasis. Testimonials tend to confirm this recommendation. Apparently we can heighten the effect if we apply Kombucha externally to the skin while also drinking it. Adding silica to the diet is another good step for clearing up and preventing skin disease, especially in genetically predisposed individuals. Stress seems to play a role in bringing on skin problems and if this is the case, we should remove the source of the stress. Meanwhile, increasing your intake of the B vitamins will help to manage stress.

Rheumatism:

Writer and researcher Harald W. Tietze reports that Dr. Wiesner reached a 92% success rate using Kombucha tea to treat his trial subjects for rheumatism. He noted that his patients pain receded and that they could move limbs freely.

Sleep Disorders:

Despite established general age guidelines for sleep requirements (babies sixteen hours, seniors five hours), sleep is highly individual and variable. I find that sometimes I need twelve hours of sleep and other times I need only three. If there aren't any underlying ailments, drinking Kombucha tea just before bedtime can help overcome problems with falling asleep and not sleeping soundly.

Stomach – see Bowels

Stones:

People who do not drink enough fluids are generally prone to develop stones. For this reason, drinking Kombucha tea is already remedial because of the higher fluid intake. As well, studies have shown, drinking Kombucha reduces and dissolves stones.

Tonsillitis:

Russian researchers could reduce the inflammation of tonsillitis with Kombucha tea administration. Personally I hold that we should only surgically remove the tonsils in the most dire circumstances. My own naturopathic family doctor saved me from a tonsillectomy (my older brother had his removed) and I have always ascribed some of my resistance to infections and colds to my protective tonsils fighting off intruders. My older brother is subject to frequent colds and flu because he is minus his tonsils.

Doggone Good for Pets

After World War II, the former Soviet Union embarked on extensive research on Kombucha in veterinary use. A preparation called "Bactericidin" made from the Kombucha symbiosis was tried on dogs, sheep, calves and other mammals. Clinical trials with lambs and calves suffering from dysentery and *colibacillosis* resulted in a 100% recovery. Mixing the Kombucha preparation into chicken feed led to a 15% increase in baby chick growth. Harald W. Tietze mentions a Kombucha trial conducted on sheep and calves, in which they treated animals suffering from diarrhea with 100% success. Also, healthy animals increased 15% in growth when Kombucha was added to their feed.

Many people give Kombucha to their dogs and cats to improve their health. According to some experts, including Betsy Pryor, the tea eliminates "doggie breath" and extreme body odor. I have adopted giving Kombucha tea to my dog because he suffers the aftereffects of being hit by a car. Bing's problem involves nerve death (paresis) of the right front paw. He is showing some improvements. He drags his right fore limb considerably less than before.

In the end we yet depend on
creatures that we made.
GOETHE

Part 2

HELPER TEA CELLS

At morn I journeyed to the novel West;
I found an unknown savour in the feast
and in the casual wine an unknown zest,
that day's first dusk had led me back to East.
1001 Nights – The Tale of The Magic Book

Chapter Four

The Mushroom's Illustrious Past

Was It Sponge or Lichen Rising in the East?

As with all ancient things, we do not know exactly how or where the Kombucha originated though all signs point to the East. Chances are that the Kombucha culture originated in the Far East, probably in China. However, Kombucha researcher Betsy Pryor thinks that the mushroom may have originated in the Middle East and made its way via the Far East to Europe and America. She bases her belief on the fact that Kombucha contains some lichen (which has antibacterial usnic acid), which according to some theories, is a major constituent of manna. Described in the Bible as feeding the children of Israel, manna is known as "food from heaven." Betsy Pryor suggests that Kombucha winded its way along the traditional spice routes that existed between the Mediterranean and the Far East. Kombucha would have been a popular beverage because caravans took months to traverse great distances and they needed fermented foods that would not spoil.

However, according to author Günther Frank, the first recorded use of Kombucha tea takes us to China. In the year 221 BC, during the Tsin Dynasty, Kombucha was hailed as "the Tea of Immortality." In China it was and is still a favorite folk remedy, but just what is it?

According to Helmut Golz, the Kombucha symbiosis was initially considered a sponge. They reinforced this belief by advertising Kombucha as a sponge being fished from the sea. It followed that people ascribed the curative properties of Kombucha to the iodine content present in sponges growing in the ocean.

Around the same time, researchers from the Central Bacteriological Institute in Moscow, after investigating the Kombucha, thought it was lichen. Lichen originated some 2.5 million years ago from a symbiosis of algae and fungi. The algae joined the mushrooms to enable the algae to survive on dry land. Now, we are getting closer. Phytotherapy, the science of plant medicine, accords many healing properties to lichen and mosses, such as the Icelandic moss. Regardless of its precise composition, the Kombucha prospered under the hands of skilled healers and slowly made its way across Siberia and into Russia proper, where it still thrives as a folk remedy.

In recent times, Western science ultimately established the Kombucha to be a symbiosis of microorganisms consisting of both bacteria and yeast cells and not sponge, moss or lichen. The fact that lichens, according to researcher Frank, require light for photosynthesis, whereas the Kombucha symbiosis happily continues to grow in total darkness proves that Kombucha is not a lichen.

Was It Bacteria or Yeast Going West?

Once in Russia, the Kombucha quickly made a name for itself as a kind of kvass. Kvass is the name of a sour beerlike beverage made of rye meal and malt. The Russians made other ingredients into kvass which they often enhanced with spices. By the turn of the century, the Kombucha had travelled from Mongolia and Russia further into the West. For a brief time, Kombucha became known (and then forgotten) in Europe. In 1913, sources describe Kombucha for the first time in German literature. A Kombucha coming from Mitawa, Russia is discussed. It says, "they employed it against all kind of ailments."

The making of tea kvass was very popular. The Russian texts refer to a Japanese or Manchurian Mushroom for this kvass. From Russia, the kvass made its way into Poland at the time of the first world war. Records show a Polish apothecarian preparing a laxative based on a

"Russian secret recipe." By 1914, they had heard of Kombucha in Prague. After World War I, Kombucha made a comeback first in Denmark and then in Germany's East Prussia province. Returning prisoners of war carried the mushroom to German Stettin and into Saxony. By 1927, some people in Westphalia and Hamburg knew it as a home remedy.

Following World War II, Kombucha became known primarily in Italy, but also in France and Spain. Strangely enough, in Germany at this time, it had been forgotten. Apart from my own theory that people forgot Kombucha because of the pressing business of daily survival, we do not know why the mushroom has gone through periods of renown and relative obscurity. My theory is probably right because they rationed everything during the war years, including sugar. Who could afford to feed sugar to a symbiotic mushroom?

In Germany, Kombucha saw a renaissance through the work of Dr. Rudolf Sklenar. This medical practitioner used it extensively in his practice to treat cancer patients. (Apparently, this method was also practiced by Dr. Veronika Carstens, the wife of the former President of West Germany.) Dr. Sklenar also prescribed it for metabolic disorders, rheumatism, gout, high blood pressure, increased blood lipid values and diabetes. He recorded various successes in these areas but was particularly concerned about finding a cure for cancer because he frowned upon orthodox cancer treatments, such as surgery and chemotherapy, and preferred biological therapies for prevention and healing.

A Kombucha by Any Other Name

Given its turbulent history, there are by now many names for the mushroom and the mushroom tea. Some of these are used in English speaking countries in place of the name Kombucha. Others are used only in other languages but can help to shed light on the tea's history. To satisfy sheer curiosity, if nothing else, I have listed all the names I know for the Kombucha mushroom. Also, I have included a variety of the names given to Kombucha tea by countries around the world. This may help identify Kombucha no matter how obscure its appellation.

Algae Fungus
Algentee (German)
Brinum-Ssene (Latvian for wondrous mushroom)
Cajnyi Kvas (Russian)
Cajnyj Grib (Russian)
Chamboucho (Rumanian)
Champagne of Life
Champignon Miracle (French)
Champignon or Elixir de Longue Vie Combucha (French)
Chinapilz (German)
Chinesischer Teepilz (German)
Comboucha (French/Japanese)
CombuchagetrÑnk (German)
Divine Che
Fungojapon (former commercial name)
Fungus Japonicus (pharmaceutical name)
Fungus Tea
Funko Cinese (Italian)
Gichtqualle (German for gout jellyfish)
Gift of Life
Godly Tsche
Gout/Hero Fungus
Haipao
Heldenpilz (German for hero's mushroom)
Hongo (Spanish)
Indian Wine Fungus/Mushroom
Indisch-Japanischer Teepilz (German)
Indischer Weinpilz (German)
Indischer Teeschwamm (German)
Indischer Teepilz (German)
Japanese Fungus/Sponge
Japanische Combucha (German)
Japanischer Teepilz (German)
Japanisches Mütterchen (German)
Japanpilz (German)
Japonskij Grib (Russian)
Kargasok Teepilz (German for tea mushroom)
Kargasok Schwamm (German for sponge)
Kargasoktee (German for tea)
Kouchakinoko (Japanese for black tea/mushroom)
Kombucha Sponge/Kvass
Kombucha-Thee (Dutch)
Kombuchamost (German)
Kombuchaschwamm (German)
Kombuchawein (German)
Kongo
Kvass/Kwas
K'un-Pu-Ch'a
Ling Zhi (Chinese)
Little Japanese Mother
Ma-Gu
Magic Mushroom
Manchurian Elixir/Fungus/Sponge/Tea
Medusa Tea
Miracle Mushroom
Mo-Gñ (former commercial term)
Olinka (Bohemian)
Red Tea Fungus
Reishi (Japanese)
Russian Flower/Jellyfish
Russian Tea-Vinegar
Russische Blume (German for Russian flower)
Russische Mutter (German for Russian mother)
Te-Aramoana
Tea Fungus/Wine/Beer/Cider
Tea Mould (Javanese)
Tea Plant/Beast
Tee Kwass
Teemost (German for tea must/cider)
Teyi Saki (Armenian)
Thee-Schimmel (Dutch)
Theebier (Dutch)
Theezwam Komboecha (Dutch)
Titania
Tschambucco
Tsche of Kombu
Volga Mushroom/Jellyfish
Wunderpilz (German for wondrous mushroom)
Yaponge
Zauberpilz (German for magic mushroom)
Zaubersaft (German for magic juice)
Zaubertrank (German for magic potion)

Wow! According to Pastor Weidinger, the word Kombucha is derived from the Japanese terms "Kombu" for brown algae and "cha" for tea. Others ascribe "Kombu" to a Korean physician by the name of Kombu, who allegedly treated the Japanese Emperor Inkyo with the cultured tea as long ago as 415 AD. Something that has had so many illustrious appellations and possible origins cannot be a hoax. Kombucha must have impressed folks all over the world to have such fanciful names. That by itself is a good indication of its true worth. If it had not tasted so refreshing, if it had not worked to restore health, people would not have forgotten it, they would have discarded it forever.

Authenticating Your Kombucha Mushroom

How can we make sure we have the true tea mushroom? Where can we obtain the right tea mushroom? Well, you might have gleaned the answer already, there isn't one true mushroom. Instead there are a number of similar bacteria and yeast cultures in symbiosis that we know as Kombucha.

The existing literature has verified this view. Each different bacteria and different yeasts form slightly different symbiotic relationships. This leads to interesting differences in taste as well. Perhaps like me, you want to practice with different Kombucha mushrooms from different regions. Presently, I have two strains fermenting and they taste slightly different. But let us settle this scientifically.

Ultimately the scientific literature talks of the following main components of the symbiotic mushroom: the yeast *Schizo saccharomyces pombe* and the bacterium *Acetobacter xylinum*. According to Helmut Golz additional members of the symbiotic relationship consist of Bacterium *Acetobacter xylinoides*, *Gluconobacter bluconicum*, *Acetobacter aceti*, *Acetobacter pasteurianum* and the additional yeasts from *Apiculatus*, *Saccharomycodes ludwigii*, *Pichia* fermentans, *Mycoderma* and yeasts from *Torula*. If in doubt, have a biochemist analyze your mushroom.

Scientific Research Results

Around 1929, a research team in Prague under Dr. Siegwart Hermann used cats injected with a cholesterol-like compound to increase blood pressure and cholesterol levels and by that cause an artificial arteriosclerosis to test Kombucha's detoxifying powers.

Arteriosclerosis leads to heart attacks or strokes in humans. This is the same in cats. The test cats showed up to thirteen times normal cholesterol levels. Dr. Hermann's team found that despite this, cats whom they simultaneously fed Kombucha could tolerate the high levels. They concluded that the Kombucha administration helped the body to cope with raised cholesterol and blood pressure levels. However, such data does not necessarily apply to human responses.

The team also tested the effects of gluconic acid (a constituent of fermented Kombucha tea) and found that phosphate stones (bladder stones) were dissolved *in vitro* and approximated by *in vivo* tests on rabbits. (Again we cannot directly apply the data to humans.) In Russia, tests done with Kombucha tincture successfully treated infections of the cornea of rabbits. Similar treatment of human conjunctivitis was equally successful. The University Clinic of Moscow successfully healed stomatitis in toddlers within five days by drinking and rinsing their mouths out with Kombucha tea.

In Omsk, they treated babies suffering dysentery exclusively with Kombucha. After one week of therapy, symptoms receded and dysentery bacteria could not be found in the stool. Again in Omsk, patients with purulent tonsillitis were treated. The treatment entailed gargling up to ten times a day with Kombucha tea and doing mouth rinses for up to fifteen minutes. The tonsillitis cleared up and even some chronic paranasal sinusitis and bowel ailments improved. The same clinic treated high blood pressure (hypertension) and arteriosclerosis with Kombucha tea. After up to three weeks, the clinic recorded an improvement in symptoms and a noticeable lowering of the cholesterol levels.

In Moscow, further tests done with mice showed that they could stimulate certain antibacterial factors and by that activate the immune system. Animals that were fed the Kombucha extract twenty-four hours before being exposed to a bacterial infection had an 80% higher survival rate than a control group. Other tests showed a stimulative effect on the pituitary-adrenal cortex systems.

Author Frank tells us that by 1914, researcher Bacinskaya found the beverage effective in regulating the intestinal tract. To tone the activity of the intestines, Frank recommends drinking a small glass of Kombucha beverage before each meal and gradually increasing this amount. Also, Frank says that in 1917, Professor Rudolf Kobert, a Privy Councillor, recalled an infallible cure for rheumatism prepared from the Kombucha culture. Also, Professor Wilhelm Henneberg found the Russian kvass to combat "all kinds of illness, especially constipation."

In 1927, Dr. Madaus writes in *Biological Method of Healing* that the Kombucha culture and its metabolic products affect the regeneration of cell walls and is therefore an excellent remedy for "hardening of the arteries." According to Tom Valentine, in 1928 Dr. Maxim Bing found the Kombucha a "very effective means of combatting hardening of the arteries, gout and sluggishness of the bowels." Bing goes on to say that "favorable results are obtained in the kidneys and the capillary vessels of the brain." In 1929, Dr. E. Arauner confirmed that the Kombucha culture is the "most effective natural folk remedy for fatigue, nervous tension, incipient signs of old age, hardening of the arteries, sluggishness of the bowels, gout, rheumatism, hemorrhoids and diabetes."

Modern studies done by Dr. Reinhold Wiesner, a medical doctor in Schwanewede, Lower Saxony, Germany, who uses electronic bioresonator tests, showed antibiotic properties in Kombucha tea. In a comparative study with an interferon preparation, Wiesner showed that Kombucha has comparable efficacy on certain illnesses. The test involved 250 patients suffering from a variety of ailments including rheumatism, asthma and kidney diseases. The effects of Kombucha exceeded those of the interferon in the asthma cases. Wiesner sees Kombucha as a biological food with antiviral properties and without unwanted side effects.

In the Dutch magazine *Op Zoek*, a 15 year old boy recalls, "the misery began when I was ten years old, and it lasted 4 years. At first the itching began in my arms, and I scratched them till they bled, especially in bed at night. After six weeks I went to the doctor. I was given a course in penicillin and ointment, because one arm was inflamed from the scratching. This lasted for about a year and a half. I kept getting more ointment, one lot after the other and it was the same with the penicillin. Finally, I had to go to a hospital specialist. The doctor talked about some intestinal bacteria which were the cause of the trouble. Then I was given more medicine, which made me feel numb, but the itching remained . . . but now my mother's been making Kombucha tea for the past six months. I began drinking it right away, and after only one week the itching was gone. I feel as if I've been born again. Even the scars are hardly visible anymore. I'd like to tell everybody to stop taking medicine and drink Kombucha."

Fungus vs Fungus: Can Kombucha Conquer Cancer?

I believe that cancer is a systemic disease that requires a holistic approach. Orthodox medicine echoes this theory and employs many remedies simultaneously; yet, its approach is far from holistic. Kombucha has been found to play a role at least in supportive cancer therapy. Some credible researchers point out that there are not clinical studies to support the role of Kombucha in cancer therapy despite Sklenar's work.

Still, it may be worth a try to add it to cancer therapy. Writer-researcher Rosina Fasching holds that the cancer fighting properties of the Kombucha beverage are due to its ability to restore the human body's metabolism to the energetic natural state that healthy, active people of all ages enjoy.

Scientists always become prudent when sweeping cancer statements are made for either a new orthodox cancer medicine, such as interferon, or a cancer fighting food, such as red beets. What we do know is that our intestinal flora, the friendly bacteria, play an important role in displacing and destroying carcinogens. Medicine distinguishes between two forms of evaluation of the history of cancer. These are respectively called diagnosis and prognosis. I would like to emphasize the third evaluation for cancer, namely prevention.

In the Canadian edition of *How to Fight Cancer & Win*, Chapter IX explores "The Healing Power of Lactic Acid." This chapter explains how lactic acid works as a repressor of cancer cells without harm to healthy cells. (Anyone battling cancer should read this book.) Lactic acid is produced through a unique souring or fermentation process, which is how Kombucha tea is made. Medical knowledge of lactic acid fermentation and its role in prevention and healing caused a German medical doctor, Dr. Sklenar, to take a closer look at employing the Kombucha fungus in cancer therapy. Lactic acid is fermented with the help of *Lactobacillus.*

Researcher Gunter Enderlein holds that the positive microbial action of the Kombucha inside the human system has the power to destroy the carcinogenic terrain required by the cancerous growth. By cleansing the system, by restoring the intestinal flora, and by balancing the body's crucial pH balance, the Kombucha helps the body's natural immune system to regain control over proliferating cancer cells. Furthermore, Enderlein holds that a cancer enhancing microbe is the culprit for causing cancer cells to divide unnaturally and unchecked and that only natural means, such as the Kombucha drink, can effectively fight cancer.

This is strictly my personal opinion, but I happen to agree with Enderlein. The evidence of failing orthodox cancer therapies is overwhelming. I saw my own mother destroyed by cancer over a ten year period. Her treatments included surgery and chemotherapy. These treatment methods still exist, and orthodox medicine is coming up with new and more aggressive ways of employing intensive chemotherapy. Nevertheless, we have come a long way toward recognition of natural remedies in the treatment of cancer. No one is pretending that it is easy to decide a course of treatment when your life is at stake, but there is hope for alternative choices.

Witness the fact that they diagnosed Ronald Reagan, the former President of the United States, with cancer while he was holding office. His treatment became public knowledge and of great media concern. Kombucha researcher Günther Frank says that Reagan got news of the cancer fighting powers of Kombucha tea through the Nobel prize winner Aleksandr Solzhenitsyn, whom they diagnosed with cancer in 1952. According to his book *The Cancer Ward*, Solzhenitsyn conquered cancer in 1953 in the hospital in Tashkent, Russia. (Also, Solzhenitsyn says that he and others in the Gulag, the prison colony in Siberia, survived mainly due to the Kombucha tea they fermented and drank.) Reportedly, Ronald Reagan obtained a Kombucha culture from Japan and drank one liter of tea daily. Reagan's cancer was prevented from spreading. As I am writing in mid-1995, Ronald Reagan is still fulfilling some public functions. It would appear that he is free of cancer, although he is now suffering from Alzheimer's.

For a possible explanation of how cancer is overcome by Kombucha, Rosina Fasching offers, "the Kombucha fungus sprouts in an acidic environment and thus eliminates or retards in its development the primitive cancer causing microbe that thrives in an alkaline environment and thus renders it, or keeps it harmless for man. The treatment of cancer and of precancerous stages including tumors, has a simple key: fungus versus fungus!"

There is a story about Joseph Stalin, who was reportedly paranoid about getting cancer. Therefore, he encouraged research into possible cancer cures. Thus prompted, his researchers found a region in Russia that was practically void of cancer occurrences, with only a few cases from immigrants to the area (Ssolikams and Beresniki districts). Oddly enough, the area was environmentally stressed with trees and fish dying from pollution. Finally the researchers came across this region's tea kvass, served to them as a refreshing beverage. Subsequent investigation by the Central Bacteriological Institute in Moscow found this kvass to be none other than our Kombucha drink formed by the symbiotic growths of Bacterium *zylinum* and yeast cells of the genus *Saccharomyces*. It didn't help Stalin though because agents in the KGB convinced him that the doctors were "out to get him" and his physician was jailed.

Kombucha and Diabetes

Due to the sugar in Kombucha tea, a Viennese professor prepared a sugarless Kombucha in the 1920s. Administration to diabetics showed, in some cases, a noticeable lowering of the blood sugar level and, in many patients, improvement of their well-being. Professor Pal ascribed the effect to the gluconic acid present in the tea. At that time, medicine held gluconic acid in high regard because, contrary to glucose or dextrose, even the diabetic organism can burn it and use its high energy content.

Some commercially available Kombucha products contain less sugar than the tea kvass you make at home. This drink may be more suitable for diabetics even though the initially high sugar content of the tea, which serves as food for the symbiosis, is transformed during fermentation into other constituents, such as gluconic acid. By leaving the fermentation process working for a few extra days, the entire sugar content is converted. A longer fermenting time does result in a drink that is more vinegary.

The microbe is nothing. The terrain (environment) is everything!
LOUIS PASTEUR

Chapter Five

Metabolism and Maladies

A Food with a Sense of Culture

Despite the many illustrious names it carries, Kombucha is not really a mushroom in the proper biological sense. It is not an alga or even a fungus. So what do we have in Kombucha? Simply speaking, Kombucha is a culture of microorganisms "symbioting" in a medium of cellulose. It is similar to a yogurt culture that ferments in milk.

So Kombucha tea is the result of a fermentation process. The fermenting causes complex changes in the organic compound by the action of enzymes that resident microbes produce. Unlike modern chemistry, microbial fermentation is a natural process that has been around for centuries. Ancient people made yogurt and butter that way. Alcohol, too, is derived from a fermentation process by which yeast ferments grape juice into wine, barley into beer and whisky.

As we have learned, the ancients of the Far East used a culture of yeast and bacteria to make the Kombucha drink. Kombucha, mainly for the sake of convenience, is called a mushroom. It does after all "mushroom" or grow quickly, so it is aptly named. Also, people call the Kombucha a fungus because it contains yeast, yeast in symbiosis with bacteria. Now all the Candida albicans victims and experts will avoid it. However, according to Tom Valentine, Günther Frank says that the *Saccharomycodes* in Kombucha is a yeast that does not throw off spores and does therefore not belong to the Candida family.

Frank argues that it therefore can be antagonistic to the troublesome Candida albicans that plague so many people, especially women. Frank goes on to explain that "most of the *ascomycetes* such as penicillin, ergot, bread mould, mildew, thrush (Candida) and others reproduce by means of spores, most of the yeasts reproduce by means of budding (or a combination of budding and fission). The fission yeasts reproduce by fission like bacteria. They do not bud nor have spores. The fission yeast in the Kombucha culture belongs to this type." Note: Drinking Kombucha tea as a remedy for Candida is not advisable without guidance from a naturopath.

Acid, Alkaline and Neutral pH

Researcher Frank also reports that "acids have a preservative effect in that they produce in the foodstuffs to be preserved a pH value which certain microbes can no longer tolerate, in particular those which create toxins. To a certain extent the Kombucha beverage preserves itself. Any alien organisms are repressed through the acids it produces." The pH in Kombucha tea is important. It varies from 2.8 to 4. When it tastes like cider, Kombucha has a pH reading of about 3.0.

The pH, the abbreviation for potential of hydrogen, sets numerical values to acid-base balances. The acidity and alkalinity of a substance is called its pH. A substance that is neutral, neither alkaline or acidic, has a pH of seven. A number below seven indicates an acid pH and a number above seven indicates an alkaline pH. For instance, the pH of the gastric juices in the stomach is normally quite acidic, between 1.0 and 5.0. While, the pH of the blood plasma is quite alkaline, between 7.35 and 7.45. Each pH step from 0 to 14 indicates a tenfold increase in pH. In healthy people the action of buffer systems of the blood and the regulatory functions of the respiratory and urinary systems holds all body fluids in equilibrium. Acidosis describes a state of excessive acidity in body fluids and alkalosis, excessive alkalinity.The body's pH balance is crucial to the maintenance of overall health.

Balancing Your Body's Hydrogen Potential

It is interesting (and noteworthy for anyone interested in pursuing longevity) that young people have a lower pH reading than older people. In other words, pH readings tend to increase with age when the blood becomes more alkaline. Normally the balance of the pH is kept in a strict equilibrium by the autonomous system that reacts quickly to offset any disturbance in pH, either by calling on calcium reserves to increase alkalinity or by liberating hydrogen ions (called protons) to increase acidity. So we do not really need to concern ourselves with our pH, or do we?

Natural healers hold that acid foods (most fruit) increase alkalinity and alkaline foods (milk, bananas) increase acidity. So you can take indirect control over your body's pH by controlling your food intake according to your pH balancing needs. If, for instance, you suffer from an upset stomach due to hyperacidity, you may benefit from eating a sour fruit such as an apple.

This may be opposite to conventional wisdom, but when suffering from stomach acidosis, usually due to incorrect eating, eat a sour fruit. Relief is almost as instantaneous as with taking in an alkaline substance such as milk, but with the greater long term benefit of healing the underlying imbalance rather than temporarily masking the upset. Kombucha is particularly effective in balancing the body's pH, because of its acidic nature. Could we relate a reported rejuvenating effect to the different pH values in young and old? Can Kombucha lower the pH reading on long term use and thereby cause a kind of rejuvenation? These are interesting questions yet to be answered by science.

L(+) vs D(-) Lactic Acid: What's All the Fuss About?

The production of lactic acid is a natural part of the active human metabolism. The friendly *Lactobacillus* such as *acidophilus*, *bulgaricus* and kefir used in making yogurt and other cultured milk products produce lactic acid in the fermentation process. Unlike alcohol fermentation, lactic acid fermentation can be defined as a living process that doesn't kill the hard working microbes. Lactic acid fermentation always creates new bacteria.

It is a major means of natural preservation of foods such as cheeses and sauerkraut. There are two kinds of lactic acids: the good L(+) lactic acid and the bad D(-) lactic acid. L(+) lactic acid, assists the circulation of the blood, and prevents decay in the bowels and constipation by promoting bowel movements. It maintains the balance between acids and alkalines. Its rich vitamin C content supports the body's natural resistance against infections and assists and encourages the function of the pancreas which in turn stimulates the secretions of all the digestive organs. D(-) lactic acid, on the other hand, is a foreign substance that enters the body through food intake and through overexertion of muscles. Cancer cells also contain D(-) lactic acid which is produced due to lack of oxygen. Blood, muscle and the stomach contain the good lactic acid L(+). Certain bacteria produce D(-) lactic acid. Fermented foods contain both kinds of lactic acid, but usually more of the L(+) lactic acid. The higher the L(+) content of a lactic acid, the better its enzymatic value for the human metabolism. Kombucha produces primarily L(+) lactic acid, which according to cancer authority Dr. Johannes Kuhl (mentioned in *How to Fight Cancer & Win*), "prevents chronic conditions from developing if taken regularly. In disease that is already encysted (established) it can effect a specific healing and protective action."

Gluconic and Glucuronic Acids and the B Vitamins in Kombucha

Gluconic acid results from the incomplete oxidation of glucose (sugar) and is a product that results from fermenting Kombucha. Gluconic acid is important to the body's utilization of metallic minerals such as calcium. Though many researchers report large quantities of glucuronic acid in the fermented beverage, author and botanist Christopher Hobbs says this is impossible. He says that, "no credible laboratory analysis of Kombucha tea has found glucuronic acid." Yet, according to ProNatura, the Dr. Sklenar formula for Kombucha tea contains glucuronic acid. As well, researcher Betsy Pryor says that both the FDA and the State of California confirm that properly prepared Kombucha tea contains glucuronic acid.

Why all the fuss? Well, glucuronic acid is a metabolite that a healthy liver produces. Glucuronic acid is vital to the detoxification process of the body. The glucuronic acid binds metabolic and environmental toxins and poisons and then excretes them. Once bound to glucuronic acid, the body cannot resorb the toxins into its tissues. According to author Günther Frank, this detoxification process is responsible for healing gout, rheumatism and arthritis because the offending toxins are flushed out through the urine in the bound up form of glucuronides or conjugated glucuronic acids.

Glucuronic acid is a precursor for mucopolysaccharide. Known also as glycosaminoglycans, these mucopolysaccharides are key tissue constituents that bond with water and are necessary in many places in the body. They are important to the prevention of wrinkling of the skin because the colloidal connective tissues underlying the skin are responsible for retaining firmness of the skin. This has an implication for many gelatinous tissues in the body and may account for the broad range of benefits from drinking Kombucha. There are mixed reports about the major ingredients found in fermented Kombucha tea, so I will list them in the following chart.

List of Ingredients:

1. Acetic acid; detoxifying
2. Carbonic acid
3. Cobalamin, cyanocobalamin (Vitamin B12)
4. Enzymes; various
5. Folic acid
6. Gluconic acid; from glucose, used in food preservation
7. Glucuronic acid

   Claim: According to Kurt Kloos of ProNatura and Kombucha researcher Betsy Pryor (and the FDA and State of California), glucuronic acid is contained in the bacterial symbiotes that make up the Kombucha. Glucuronic acid occurs only in fauna (animals) and not in flora (plants).

   Counterclaim: According to Christopher Hobbs, glucuronic acid is not contained in Kombucha. However, green tea (the base for black tea) can prompt the liver to manufacture glucuronic acid.
8. Lactic acid; mildly detoxifying
9. Niacin, niacinamide (Vitamin B3)
10. Pyridoxine (Vitamin B6)
11. Riboflavin (Vitamin B2)
12. Thiamine (Vitamin B1)
13. Usnic acid

    Claim: This is a lichen acid, which according to some experts is found in Kombucha.

    Counterclaim: This is denied by author Christopher Hobbs, who claims to have researched this thoroughly.
14. Other acids possibly present: Hydroxy acid: (citric acid, tartaric acid, succinic acid, malonic acid, oxalic acid); Amino acids: (lysine, alanine, tyrosine, valine, phenylalanine, leucine, isoleucine, aspartic acid, glutamic acid, serine, threonine)

Perhaps an easier way of assessing this would be to ask yourself if your liver is up to snuff. If you have a history of smoking, frequent use of commercial antibiotics, pharmaceuticals and/or drug addiction, alcohol abuse or excessive junk food eating, your overtaxed liver could use help. Kombucha tea seems to hold one key to accelerated detoxification of the body because other than the liver and Kombucha, glucuronic acid cannot be found in nature. As a pleasant side effect of the glucuronic acid in the tea, you will feel energized because a toxic liver may be the primary cause of chronic fatigue. Combine Kombucha tea drinking with milk thistle treatment and you may feel rejuvenated twice as fast.

Through their own metabolic activities microorganisms produce a number of useful substances, such as the B vitamins, acids and enzymes listed in the previous chart. Moreover, according to Hobbs, many volatile compounds occur to impart characteristic sweet, sour flavors and smells. (diacetyl, acetoin, isobutyraldehyde, vanillic acid, anisaldehyde, valeraldehyde, methyllisobutyl ketone, esters of methyl, ethyl, isobutyl, isoamyl alcohols).

Externally Yours: Compresses, Wounds, Ulcers, Beauty and Bath Aids

Other Kombucha books report people's successes with Kombucha compresses as well as taking the tea internally for preventing wrinkles and clearing up skin problems. For purposes of applying the mushroom itself, running it through your kitchen mixer can make it into a useful cream in seconds. Then with the help of a naturopath, go ahead and experiment by dressing skin conditions.

If you want an overall body treatment, add a batch of harvested Kombucha tea to your next bath. Also, apparently users have had great results from Kombucha hair packs. Researcher Fasching reports that "with elderly people Kombucha has a rejuvenating effect, causing hair to grow in dark again, tightening the skin . . . keep the teeth healthy."

One of the earliest systems of classification consisted of two kingdoms, plants and animals. Although this classification lasted a long time, it was not satisfactory because some organisms did not fit well in either kingdom.

SYMBIOSIS

Part 3

TEA CEREMONY

Ingredients & Tools

- Kombucha Mushroom
- Orange Pekoe Tea
- Refined White Sugar
- Purified Water
- Funnel
- Stainless Steel Pot
- Large Glass Bowl or Dish
- Glass Storage Containers
- Wooden or Ceramic Spoon
- White Cotton Towel or Cheesecloth

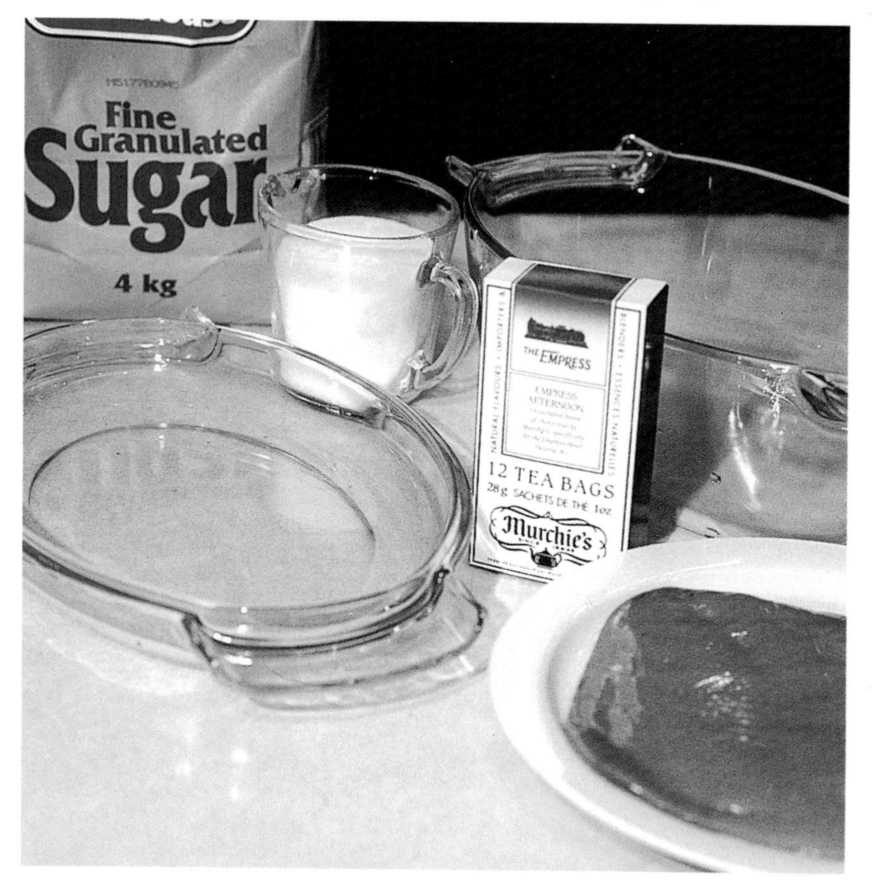

▼ The key ingredients

The tea ceremony: Making the tea and sugar solution

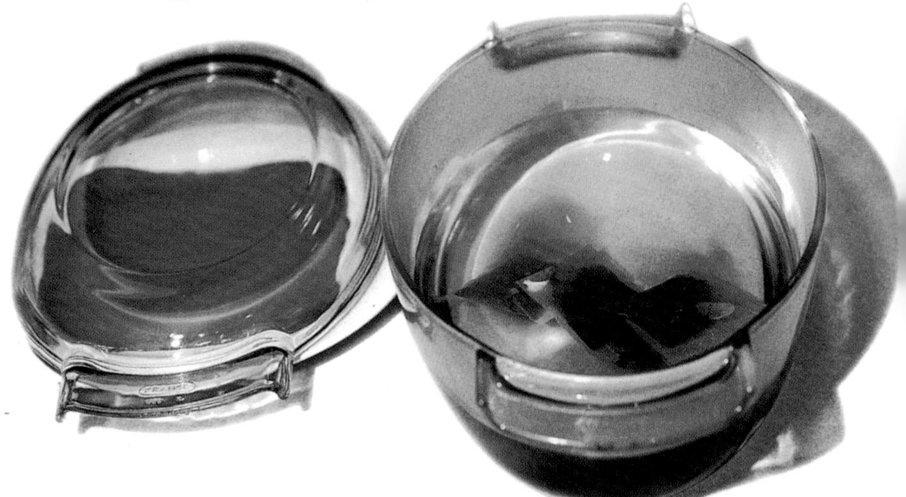

Let the tea cool to lukewarm before adding your Kombucha mushroom

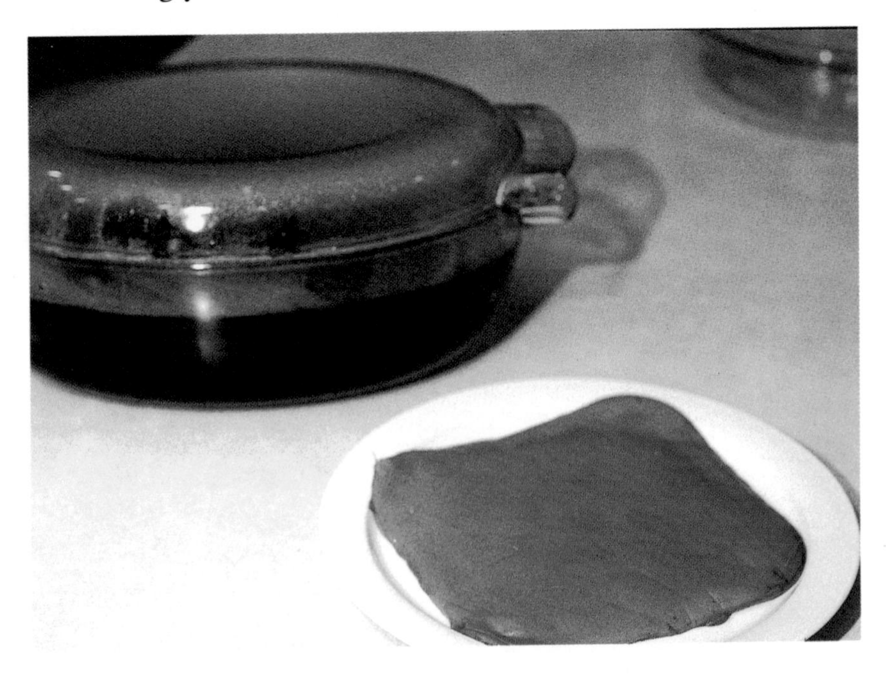

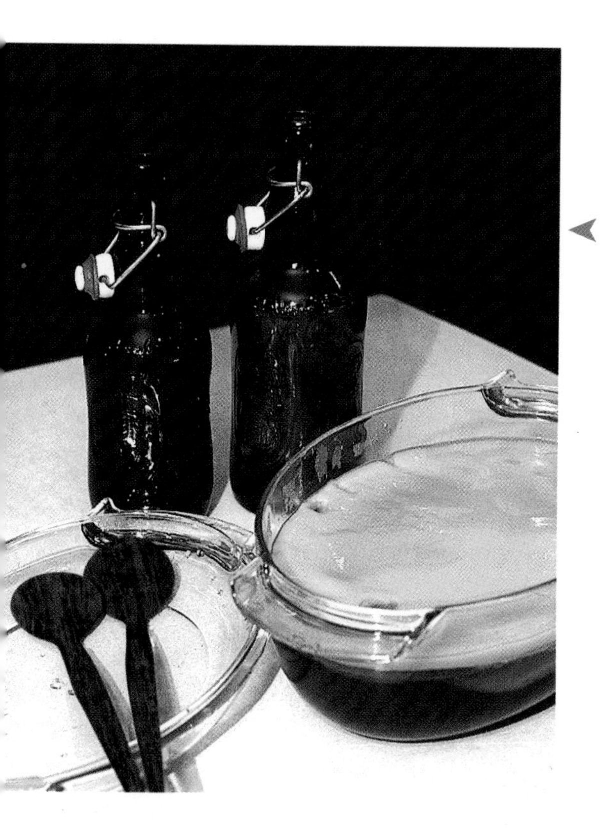

The fermenting process: The mushroom converts the sugar and tea into a variety of enzymes, acids and vitamins

Take a look at your baby Kombucha

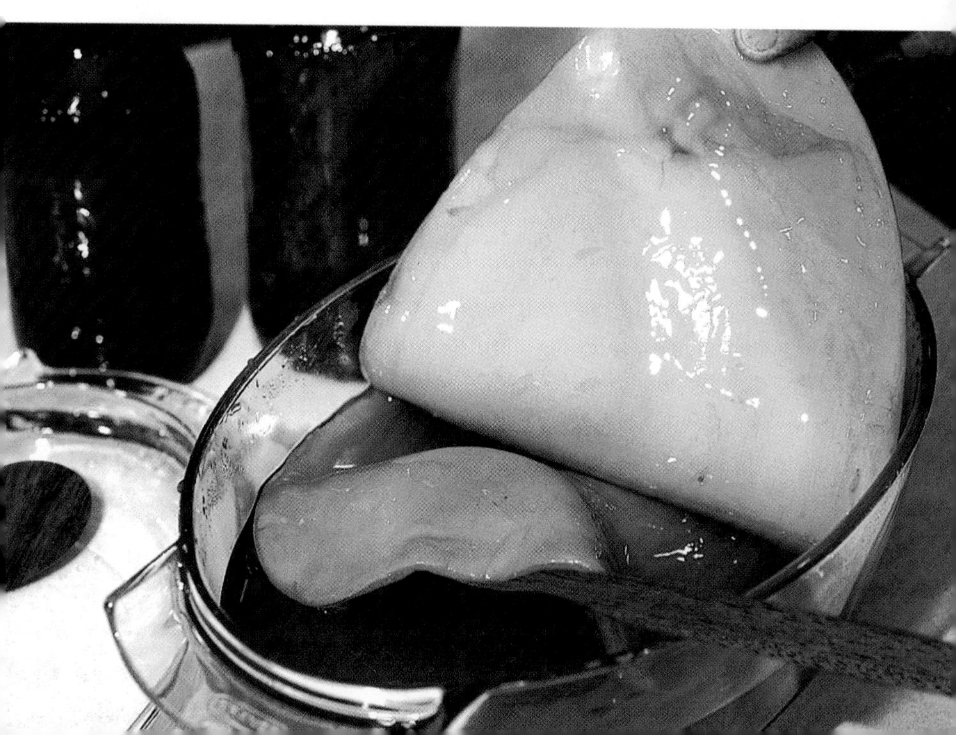

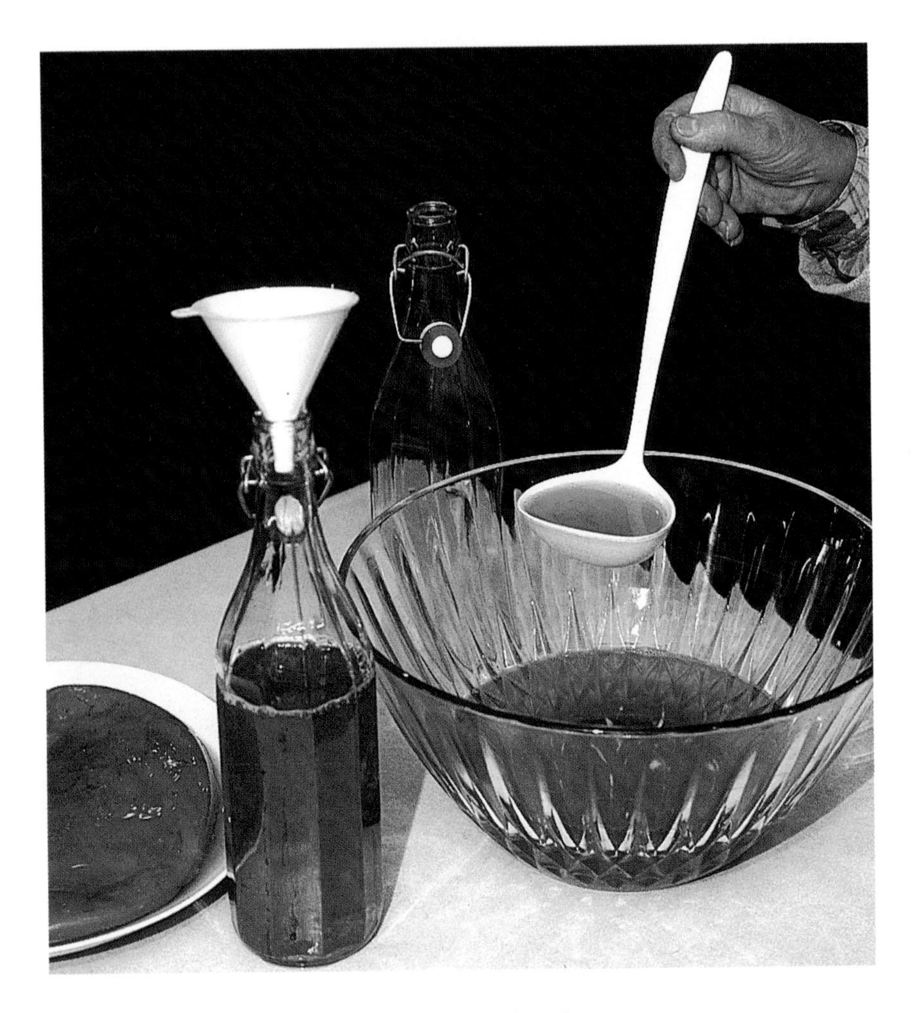

Harvesting Kombucha tea:
It's time to enjoy the delicious healing drink

Physicians are many in title
but very few in reality.
HIPPOCRATES (BC 460-370)

Chapter Six

Making Kombucha Tea

Getting Baby Home

In any successful tea ceremony, time is of the essence. "Never rush a tea ceremony," my mother told me ages ago. How much time does it take to brew Kombucha tea? Roughly speaking, it will take about thirty minutes to brew and a few minutes to cool off. Since, you are eager to start your own batch of Kombucha tea, you will want to know where you can get your own baby Kombucha. Perhaps a relative, friend or neighbor has just given you one? If not, see the Resources section.

If this is your first Kombucha mushroom, you will notice that it looks like a pancake: flat, serrated and golden brown. On touching it though, you will notice that it feels more like a rubbery pancake dipped in oil. Remember that cleanliness is essential for handling your Kombucha baby. So before you touch the new Kombucha baby (it will in all likelihood reach you in a sealed plastic pouch swimming in some of its nourishing tea), make sure your hands are clean.

The Kombucha cannot tolerate any metal, so you must remove all rings and jewelry from fingers and wrists. Wash your hands with soap and be sure to rinse all soapy residues off your fingers. Wearing clean rubber gloves is an option for people. I enjoy being in contact with the mushroom because, although cleanliness is important, complete sterile conditions are not necessary as the mushroom symbiosis will destroy intruding organisms during its fermentation cycle.

Before you concentrate on brewing the tea, you should remove the mushroom from the plastic pouch. Gently lay it in a shallow glass dish in the tea with which it came (though glass is always best, glazed ceramic or porcelain will do for this brief span). Cover it with a white cotton cloth or towel without touching the mushroom and, voila, we are ready to make tea. If for some reason you get called away during your tea ceremony, wash your hands again before touching your Kombucha mushroom.

Note: A Pyrex glass dish with lid is the best container. Remember that these dishes are ovenware only and cannot be used to boil the water. A friend of mine did this the other day. He followed the proper directions except he boiled water in his Pyrex container. When he had finished brewing his tea, he went to another room while he waited for the tea to cool. Within minutes, he heard his daughter cry out from the kitchen, "Papa! Papa! Come quickly, your Kombucha!" On entering the kitchen he found his glass container broken and his tea all over the stove and dripping on the floor. The moral is don't use a Pyrex glass dish on a burner. My friend's burst in a reaction to the heat. So use a stainless steel pot for that part of the tea-making.

What You Will Need:

It is simple to brew Kombucha tea. However, like the brewing of other teas, you must be prepared for the ceremony. Possibly, you are already prepared. Go ahead and check your kitchen cupboards. Other than a Kombucha mushroom, here is a list of things you will need to make Kombucha tea successfully.

1. Purified water:
You will need two to four liters, depending on the size of your fermenting glass bowl. Be sure to use only purified water free of silt, chlorine, metal residues from the water pipes, chemicals such as fluorine or any other toxins. Any distilled water will do as well.

2. A stainless steel pot:
This pot should hold at least 4 liters, more if possible. If you want to make more than one batch, I recommend a commercial-sized pot. Any restaurant supplier in your town will have those in stock. Look in the Yellow Pages under "Restaurant Equipment" or "Food Processing Equipment." Remember, the pot will only contain the tea, never the mushroom.

3. White sugar:
One cup depending on size of the bowl used. A rule of thumb is 1/2 cup of sugar per liter of tea. The white sugar can be refined from cane or beet sugar.

4. Black tea:
Three to five teaspoons of orange pekoe or three to five tea bags depending on quantity of tea made. I recommend using Twinings Orange Pekoe tea.

5. A large glass bowl:
You must use a glass bowl or container (three or five liter glass bowl is ideal) without any metal or plastic components, not even the rim. Plastic, ceramic or crystal will not work because of permeation problems during fermentation. The fermenting mushroom will leach impurities from plastics, ceramics and crystals. Tempered glass is good. Use a two, three or five liter Pyrex or FireKing measuring bowl. It must have a large opening for the mushroom to unfold and receive more oxygen.

6. A wooden, ceramic or glass spoon:
To stir the tea and remove the tea bags after steeping is completed.

7. A white cotton towel:
This is used to cover your Kombucha during fermentation to protect it against invading insects and dust. Any other clean white or light colored cotton towel or cloth will do, as will cheesecloth. If you do not have a cotton tea strainer, a cheesecloth or cotton towel can also serve as strainer when pouring your fermented tea into glass bottles for storage in your refrigerator.

8. A funnel:
You may need this to pour the fermented tea into the glass bottles. I simply pour my finished tea through a cotton tea strainer. If you do not have one, using a plastic funnel is fine because the tea will only pass through it very quickly. There is little chance of leaching from the plastic from such brief contact. Remember, *no metal.*

9. Glass storage containers:
These should be clear, sterile glass jars with a cork or plastic lid. Depending on the size of your batch, you will need enough of them to hold your fermented tea. Corked clear glass bottles are fine. Just make sure the lid or cork can yield to fermenting pressure for the tea will likely continue to ferment in the storage container.

Instructions:

Brewing Kombucha tea is not an exact science. Variations in taste and appearance will occur because of the uniqueness of each Kombucha mushroom and the subtle differences in your preparation methods. Though a Kombucha is "alive" and needs to be treated with care, it is quite robust and can tolerate regular handling. Try to follow these instructions as closely as possible, but remember to have fun.

Step 1: Ready to brew your tea? Pour water into a steel pot and bring to a boil. Remove the pot from the heat. Add the required amount of sugar (rule of thumb is 1/2 cup per 1 liter). Stir until the sugar completely dissolves. Alternatively, you may want to return the pot to the heat source and boil it for a few minutes with the dissolved sugar. Either method will work. I decided to begin with only 2 liters of water for my first Kombucha experience. I highly recommend this to beginners because it is easier to handle and will give you increased confidence. Also, 2 liter glass storage containers are easier to find.

Step 2: Now you add the tea. You can either make the tea in a heat-proof glass dish or in the pot. I use only Orange Pekoe tea because I found it made the tastiest tea. But if you have a favorite, you can definitely use your blend of black tea. I use and recommend Twinings tea bags. Use 5 tea bags for every 3 liters of water. Vary according to taste. Now we need some time for the infusion to complete. The recommended steeping time is 10 to 15 minutes. Steeping time for loose tea leaves is usually a bit shorter than for tea bags. You may prefer using loose or bulk packed Orange Pekoe tea. That is provided you strain the tea leaves completely after filtering the brew through a fine sieve or strainer. This clears the tea of leaf residues. If you are a beginner, I would advise you to stick with the tried and tested Orange Pekoe tea bags.

Step 3: Completed your infusion? Remove the tea bags or strain the tea leaves through a sieve, strainer, cheesecloth or cotton cloth. Cover the pot or glass dish, if you have already poured the strained tea into a heat-proof glass dish, then let it cool to lukewarm. When the tea is lukewarm, it is time to take about 8 teaspoons or up to 1/2 cup from the previous batch (or the tea that your first mushroom came in) and pour it gently into the cooled down tea. Always wait for a few extra minutes for the hot tea to cool before pouring it into the waiting glass dish or dishes, unless these are Pyrex or similar heat-proof glassware. It pays to be patient.

STEP 4: Once the lukewarm tea is in a glass container, you can take the entire Kombucha mushroom from its holding container and gently float it on top of the tea (the darker, rougher side down, the lighter, smoother side facing up). It will float nicely on top. Don't worry if some tea laps over the top. It is time for the fermenting phase.

STEP 5: Place the dish or dishes high up on a shelf in a clean area that is not far from ventilation. Wherever you undertake the fermentation process, be sure to avoid direct sunlight and the vicinity of wet, mildewy or moldy areas such as wet walls or potted plants. You do not want to the fermenting Kombucha to attract spores.

STEP 6: Wait seven to fourteen days while your Kombucha mushroom is quietly ripening. The usual fermenting time is between seven and ten days, depending on desired flavor and sugar content. A shorter fermenting period results in a sweeter tea with a higher sugar content. A longer fermenting period results in a more vinegary tea with little or no sugar.

STEP 7: It is time to remove the fermented tea from the storage shelf. Perhaps you want to peek under the cover to see the new mushroom in the dim light of your basement. Is it doing fine? Has it given birth to a baby mushroom?

STEP 8: After eight to fourteen days gently remove the covering cotton towel and carry your new harvest into the kitchen. Using your clean hands, gently separate the parent Kombucha from the baby. You now have two cultures and can double your efforts.

STEP 9: Your harvested Kombucha drink should be poured into and then stored in glass bottles that can be corked or otherwise loosely covered. It is important not to use tightly sealing glass bottles because the ferment could create enough pressure to cause a problem. You don't want to burst your bubbly! Once in a proper glass container in your fridge, the Kombucha drink will be good for a few weeks. Then, you are ready to brew your next batch of tea.

Note: Always save a cup of your latest batch for your next batch.

Why Orange Pekoe Kombucha Tea?

According to experts, tea is necessary for the Kombucha culture as it provides needed mineral salts and nitrogen, and stimulates the microorganism to grow. Tea also tastes good. People who are concerned about the caffeine in black tea should keep in mind that green tea also contains caffeine. Herbal teas contain alkaloids that might affect the Kombucha. In any event, I think that expertise in herbs is definitely necessary before embarking on trials with herbal teas and Kombucha. However, suppose that you have successfully completed your first Kombucha cycle and your original mushroom has successfully given birth to a new baby. You are an expert by now. You may want to experiment with other black teas, green teas or herbal teas. Feel free to experiment, keeping in mind that steeping time for herbal tea is less than for black tea, about half as long.

How Sweet It Is: Sugar, Honey or Saccharin

At a recent Kombucha seminar, an attendee stated, "I reasoned out...you should use raw sugar (instead of refined white sugar) because you don't have the elements that you would have in a raw sugar." He then emphasized, "which, of course, you find in molasses...one of the great foods in the world. So I throw a little molasses into mine, and I find that the rate of reaction from this approximately three times faster in forming the drink." Then, the lecturer, Betsy Pryor, told the audience that though there are ingredients that will prompt the Kombucha to ferment faster (peptone, honey, raw sugar) research conducted in Russia confirmed that refined white sugar makes the most active type of Kombucha because it has little nutritional value except as a food for the Kombucha symbiotes.

I know how tough it is to sell refined sugar to health conscious people. However, remember that the sugary solution is to feed the yeast cells and the bacterial culture only and not you. By the time you drink the Kombucha, there is little if any sugar left in the drink. The yeast and bacteria have consumed it and through their metabolic activity turned it into healthy compounds. To be more precise, according to Günther Frank, "after normal fermentation period of 14 days only three grams of simple sugars (monosaccharides) per

100 grams of Kombucha tea remain in the drink." Compare that to the seven teaspoons of sugar present in one serving of a carbonated cola.

Even so, some people recommend the use of honey as an alternative to refined sugar. However, honey contains enzymes and natural antibiotics added by the bees and these ingredients may interfere with the microbiology of your Kombucha. Most Kombucha experts agree that honey can create problems, so I would not experiment. If you want to use honey, do not add it to the boiling water, but wait until your tea has cooled down. In the end, I still recommend refined white sugar, especially to beginners to Kombucha tea-making.

Thinking about using a sugar substitute to avoid refined white sugar? Think again, because the Kombucha culture can only eat sugar as its food, no artificial sweetener will serve. The culture would starve on saccharin made from toluene, a substance that does not have any food value. If you think you can escape the refined white sugar by using brown sugar, remember that brown sugar, for the most part, is made by adding molasses to refined white sugar. Also, Frank confirms that white sugar works best for the culture. Within limits, the sweetness of the finished Kombucha drink can be controlled by the amount of sugar and the length of fermentation. Experimentation will soon let you decide the right combination for your particular tastes and needs.

If you still feel you need to avoid sugar, you may follow the advice of Dr. Meixner, who according to author Tietze, substitutes manna for sugar. Manna is not nearly as sweet as sugar, so Dr. Meixner recommends using three times more manna than sugar. Of course, he makes his own manna. If you are up to it and into travelling, I can tell where to find manna. It is a dried sweet secretion obtained from cutting into the bark of European ash shrubs and trees, especially the flowering ash at home in southern Europe (*Fraxinus ornus* and *Fraxinus rotundifolia*). Bon voyage!

Being Cool

Prematurely placing the mushroom into tea that has not cooled to room temperature may damage or even kill it. Depending on ambient temperature, season and climate, the cooling off period may take from a few minutes to several hours.

Why Must You Use Glass Dishes Only?

I happened to be watching TV in the fall of 1994. A fascinating but grisly TV special on the evils of our plastic society was aired on the CBC's *Witness* program, titled "Sex Under Siege." The solidly researched program drives home the dangers of estrogenic compounds leaching from the ordinary plastic containers that we use in our lives, especially in our kitchens, and how they endanger us and our living environment. These estrogenic compounds so closely mimic the female hormone estrogen that they are creating havoc in the hormonal household of the males of any species.

Thus, there has been a rise in boys being born with poorly developed sex organs and a simultaneous increase in hermaphroditic births. In the animal world, oil spills in the Everglades (remember that plastics are made largely from crude oil) resulted in a wipe out of all the male alligators. Only female eggs could be found. Reproduction became a problem and alligators started to disappear. Similar situations occurred with fish in the Great Lakes and in England.

So you can see why we don't want plastic dishes for our Kombucha culture which has the power to leach these dangerous compounds from material and incorporate them into their structure. I have stated elsewhere that a Kombucha cannot tolerate contact with any kind of metal. Since crystal contains a lot of lead, there is a danger of the Kombucha culture leaching lead from crystal. Since lead is highly poisonous not only to the Kombucha but also to us, that is the last thing we want. Ceramics and porcelains present similar problems in that they contain metallic elements Kombucha can't tolerate. That leaves us with using only safe, unadulterated glass made of, wouldn't you know it, the white sands of silica. So, be sure to employ only pure glass containers for fermenting and storing your Kombucha tea. Glass bottles, such as thoroughly washed wine bottles that you can cork, are great receptacles for your Kombucha drink.

How to Prepare the Tea for Fermenting

If you look at the previous glass container you used for fermenting, you will find the cup of tea I asked you to retain. At the bottom of it you will notice a bit of sediment. This is the yeast sediment left over from the fermenting process. Leave this sediment in the container which you will use again for your next batch. After you've made about three to four batches though, clean out the container by rinsing it with hot water. At that time you can throw out the yeast sediment. Leaving sediment allows you to process your next batch without having to add tea from the previous batch. Some Kombucha professionals prefer to rinse the fermenting container completely every time and adding a portion of the old tea. Both methods bring equally good results as far as I can determine.

Also, experts recommend taking the Kombucha mushroom itself at this time and rinsing it under running cold water and placing it into the fermenting container. A Kombucha does not have to be rinsed before being reused. Personally, I don't wash my Kombucha. I separate the new mushroom from the original, pour the fresh tea into clean containers, and put one cup of the old tea and the Kombucha mushroom in my glass fermenting containers.

The Right Place to Ferment

During the fermentation period, the fermenting Kombucha needs an optimal growing environment. Choose a place in your attic or basement or any other suitable room where it is not too cold or too warm. A place that is airy and away from direct sunlight is necessary. The Kombucha is best left undisturbed and in place during fermentation. I always affix a yellow sticker saying "Do Not Touch" so that unsuspecting family members will be alerted and not move the container. I successfully ferment my Kombucha in the basement, but any place in your house or apartment will do that is not in direct sunlight, has sufficient air flow, and is not hot during the day. That means that most kitchen shelves or bedrooms would qualify.

Once you have carried your mushroom covered tea in its glass container to its place of fermentation, cover it lightly with a clean white cotton towel or cloth. Now fasten the cotton around the rim of the container with a rubber band or some string to prevent the towel from touching the Kombucha and to make sure that no insects can fly in or crawl underneath the covering cloth. Having chosen the right place is as important as any of the other steps in making Kombucha tea.

How Long Should the Kombucha Ferment?

If the weather conditions are favorable, you will probably find that eight days of fermentation is ideal. If the storage area is hot, seven days may be sufficient. If the storage area is cold or you prefer a more acidic taste to the finished drink, give it ten days to ferment. After ten to fourteen days of fermenting, the sugar content is consumed entirely by the mushroom. The longer your tea ferments, the more vinegary it will taste. Don't worry if your tea accidentally ferments too long, you can use it as vinegar.

The Inside Story:

Silently in the glass container, swimming in the tea, the yeast cells of the parent mushroom are busy feeding on the nutrients provided by the sugar and the tea. As a side effect of their metabolism, they'll produce a small amount of alcohol. The proliferating yeasts create conditions under which the bacteria will begin to prosper, thereby reconverting the alcohol into acetic acid (vinegar). The yeast cells begin a decline as the bacteria grow in prominence and create enough new cellulose for a new Kombucha baby to take shape.

Incidentally, I have started one batch by using only a small portion of a Kombucha mushroom. It worked well. The fragmented Kombucha parent gave birth to a healthy, full grown baby. If for some reason you want only one mushroom for your next batch of tea and have no one to pass the second mushroom on to, you have a couple of choices. You can simply throw the old mushroom in the garbage. Better yet, you can store the old mushroom for back up and continue with the baby. Later we will explore more ways to get rid of, process, or store unwanted Kombuchas. Meanwhile, you have just graduated to minimicrobiologist. Congratulations!

No Smoking Please

We do not permit smoking of any tobacco products in our home. This is good for my Kombucha cultures because the experts have reported that tobacco smoke will interfere with successful fermentation of the Kombucha culture. So please do not let any cigarette, tobacco smoke or other noxious fumes get close to your Kombucha. For that reason I would not recommend placing the culture into your garage. If your basement is similarly affected, you must find another spot for the fermenting process. How about your attic, your kitchen or any other area where the culture can be kept warm, quiet, aired and away from direct sunlight.

Alcohol Fermentation and Kombucha Champagne

Once you have removed the mushroom floating atop, the tea will seem the same as when you first stored it away. However, you will notice that something exciting has happened when you start straining the tea from the fermenting vessel into the storage containers.

The first time I poured my Kombucha tea through a cotton cloth sieve, I was stunned. On pouring, my Kombucha tea foamed and bubbled like champagne will when opened. Except, I did not have to "open" it. It had always been exposed to air.

I just had to taste this tea. I poured myself a large glass of my newly harvested Kombucha tea from the glass carafe and with gusto, drank the whole glassful. French champagne does not taste like any other kind of bubbly. So-called champagne (in truth, we should call only bubbly from the Champagne region in France champagne) from any other place or country does not taste like French champagne. The Kombucha beverage's alcoholic content is in comparison to champagne very low; usually less than 0.5 percent. You may think you can increase the alcohol content of the tea by adding more sugar to your mixture, but that would only make your tea too acidic as the alcohol in the tea is converted into vinegar. Nevertheless, I was drinking a tea that tasted like the best drink in the world. The cost to me had been 1/2 hour of tea-making which was a fun job. By the time my wife came home to taste the drink, the foam had settled out and then we were drinking Kombucha that tasted like apple cider. Ah but, that first drink on harvest day makes it all worthwhile. In fact, if you have a large enough family, you may end up drinking all the Kombucha champagne at this time.

Hint: Starting several Kombucha ferments at two to four day intervals will give you fresh Kombucha tea every other day or every four days. This is what I am doing. I admit it's a bit more work, but if you like your tea fresh and bubbly it's worth the effort.

How to Store the Finished Tea?

The Kombucha tea minus the Kombucha mushroom will still be a little bit active and, to prevent it from fermenting further, your Kombucha beverage should be stored in a cool spot such as your refrigerator.

Multiplication Is the Name of the Game

Now, having a new baby mushroom on hand, you are ready to repeat the entire Kombucha tea ceremony. In fact, you can double up if all has gone as planned because you will have two Kombucha mushrooms to ferment. For this purpose, keep some of the freshly harvested tea. Most of the harvested tea you pour into glass bottles or carafes and store in the fridge will be consumed over the next few days and weeks. A good Kombucha program though is drinking two shot glasses full on an empty stomach every morning.

If your first batch of tea was too strong, acidy, or vinegary for your taste, you can dilute it with purified water or fresh tea. For your next batch, shorten the fermentation period or experiment with sugar content. I would not recommend experimenting unless you have more than one Kombucha.

At this point you may be wondering how many Kombucha batches you will need to ferment simultaneously to maintain a program. My own program consists of 1 cup per day per person (my wife and I drink 1/2 cup in the morning and again before retiring) and we usually have two batches fermenting. That is enough to complete our program and have some left over to pass on to family, friends and neighbors. I think you will quickly find out how much Kombucha to make depending on you and your family's needs.

Why Make Your Own Kombucha Tea?

Simply because it is one of the greatest hobbies you can have. Creating your own health lab is a fun activity and one that you can share with your loved ones. Making Kombucha tea is truly an altruistic act because you will help others by passing along the boon. Your hobby will provide you with a beverage that is healthy, delicious, inexpensive and free of preservatives.

Consider this: a German engineer recently calculated that eating just one container of prepackaged strawberry yogurt involves 9,115 km of travel for the various ingredients from the plastic to the alu-foil cover. Further information states that production and transportation of this product causes emissions of 500 kg of nitrogen oxide, 35 kg of black carbon (soot) and 32.5 kg of sulphur dioxide.

Can I Eat a Kombucha?

Why not? After all, it is made up of the same ingredients as what is dissolved in the tea, only in concentrated form. Apparently some people have eaten it and benefited, but why bother. In that condensed form it contains a lot of cellulose which the human body cannot metabolize and it probably doesn't taste pleasant. Personally, I cannot imagine eating the mushroom itself, at least not in that form.

The mushroom is the medium through which you obtain your Kombucha champagne, beer, cider, tea, drink or whatever you call your beverage. A Kombucha is supposed to be your friend for life, not for lunch.

Can I Dry a Kombucha?

This is apparently possible and ideal for shipping purposes. I haven't tried it, but Harald Tietze reports that it should be dried at 33° C (92° F) avoiding direct sunlight. Microwave ovens should never be used as they will kill the fungus. If you want to dry your Kombucha, you are probably best advised to purchase a professional dehydrator.

To regenerate the dried fungus, it should be started with a tea batch according to the following formula: 1/2 liter water, 80 g sugar, 2 tea bags and 1 teaspoon of boiled vinegar. Otherwise prepare as usual except that the fermentation period should be for at least 15 days for the first batch from the dried mushroom.

The Longevity of a Kombucha

Essentially a healthy Kombucha symbiosis lives a long life provided it is allowed to ferment under ideal conditions. (Keep out of direct sunlight but in an area with lots of oxygen.) Kombucha came down to us from uncountable generations of predecessors. So if treated correctly, the mushroom will not die. Yet, I seemed to notice that the longer a Kombucha mushroom lives and produces baby mushrooms it appears to grow old and weary. Once you're familiar with your Kombucha, you'll recognize the telltale signs of age.

This is also the case if it is kept inactive for too long either in the fridge or in an area with little air. It will start to look frazzled, spotty and dark. Do we need to look further into the life span of a Kombucha? No, I do not think so because if all has gone well, you will have so many baby Kombuchas that you can safely throw your aging Kombucha away. It has served its purpose and outlived its usefulness.

From all the expert evidence gathered to date, it appears conclusive that each baby Kombucha has the same potency as its parent. So, without further ado, go ahead and use the baby Kombucha for your next batch of tea.

What to Do When a Kombucha Goes Moldy

Sometimes mold will form on top of a fermenting Kombucha. This happened to me once. In a trial, I had mixed two different Kombuchas. I harvested this very large batch with two other batches. While the other two were fine, the mixed batch had greyish green mold spots on top of the otherwise fully developed mushroom. During the fermenting process, the bowl was not as tightly sealed as the other two batches. Perhaps this was the cause of the mold or was it the unusual mixing? I do not know.

If this happens to you, this is what you should do. You can safely wash the mold off and continue as usual. Some authors suggest washing the mother Kombucha under cold water and removing all signs of mold. After that, you must rinse it in pure apple cider vinegar. This cleansing treatment should fully restore the health of the Kombucha mushroom and make it ready for the next batch of tea.

However, I prefer to be cautious and advise my readers to be the same. When in doubt, throw it out. I trashed the entire batch. While most molds are harmless, some may be dangerous and I was not taking any chances. Follow my lead: if you see mold on your mushroom, dump it and start fresh with a new Kombucha.

What to Do When a Kombucha Dies

Chances are that your Kombucha, if it dies, has been starved to death from being deprived of sugar or slowly killed by antibiotic ingredients in honey. For this reason, no less than 50g sugar per liter of tea (or 2 ounces sugar to 1 quart tea) should be used. Your Kombucha may have been exposed to nicotine from some form of tobacco. According to Harald Tietze, this is the case in 50% of Kombucha deaths.

If your Kombucha has died and you don't have another one to keep you going, return to the source where you got your first Kombucha mushroom. If that is not possible, please refer to the Resources section in the back of this book for further guidance. Whatever it takes, we will put you back in Kombucha business.

To prevent being stuck in the first place with only a dead Kombucha mushroom you may want to store another living Kombucha mushroom, one of your babies, in the refrigerator. Kept cold, it can be sealed floating in some of its tea. Over time (3 - 6 months) this Kombucha mushroom will turn the tea into vinegar. When using this vinegary Kombucha mushroom, total fermentation time will be less because a baby mushroom will be grown quicker than ever.

Though some advise against freezing because of possible crystallization damage to the mushroom, there are reports of people having successfully stored Kombucha cultures in their freezers for up to five years, so you could always give that a try. If you have such thoughts, perhaps you should pass babies on and get one back when the time is right. You may also want to use commercial Kombucha drinks, extracts or tinctures.

A Final Caution: Never discard a Kombucha you do not need or want into your sink or toilet. It may attach somewhere and grow, eventually clogging up your drain pipes.

At mealtime come thou hither, and eat of the bread,
and dip thy morsel in the vinegar.
Ruth, 2:14

Chapter Seven

A Spoonful of Sugar

The Professional Brew

Tea rituals, you say, are not your style and the kitchen not your favorite place? Relax. You can still benefit from Kombucha. Various experts have commercially prepared a Kombucha extract and tea. They found that the Kombucha could be dried without losing its viability. However, it seems that the vitality of dried Kombucha diminishes with time. At some point it loses its ability to ferment in the sugared tea.

Today Kombucha extracts, tinctures and drinks are available in apothecaries and health food stores. The pure pressed extract is a biological medicine with a validity of its own. While the Kombucha tea is a fermentation of the Kombucha symbiosis, the pressed extract is the symbiosis itself. Thus, extracts do not employ the metabolic products of the Kombucha culture but the culture directly. Helmut Golz reports that these tinctures help heal infections with or without fevers, diverse metabolic disorders, allergic reactions, sleeplessness, fatigue and debility. The tinctures are apparently good for three months and can easily be self-administered.

If you are still concerned about the sugar content in Kombucha you may prefer some of the commercially brewed teas that give you less sugar or controlled sugar values listed on the product. If this is a route you wish to explore, check with your local health food store. Professional brews may also offer you new and exciting flavors.

A reliable Kombucha product distributor is **ProNatura**. You can find their address in the Resources section at the back of this book. The folks at ProNatura would be happy to refer you to a store in your hometown where you can purchase professional Kombucha made according to Dr. Sklenar's formula. Dr. Sklenar has been working with Kombucha for more than forty years and is considered the authority on Kombucha. The Kombucha kvass, made according to this medical doctor's formula, is considered safe. According to Kurt Kloos of ProNatura, in the more than twenty years during which they have sold his Kombucha teas and extracts in Germany there has never been a safety problem.

Kurt assures his customers that the Sklenar products taste good as well. Kombucha lover Betsy Pryor echoes this comment. She describes the Sklenar tea as delicious and confirms that ProNatura's Kombucha tea is "alive." What she means is that it is grown according to the traditional Russian formula which retains the capacity for the best fermentation.

The Philosopher's Yin-Yang

Though not a miracle healer, the Kombucha culture has the respect of Dr. Kuni Fann, a philosophy professor at York University in Toronto, Ontario. Dr. Fann, who teaches several courses on philosophy including the philosophy of languages, is currently on a sabbatical and travelling in Japan, China and Taiwan in search of scientific findings on Kombucha.

I met Dr. Fann when he was the President of Yin-Yang Natural Products and a member of the CHFA (Canadian Health Food Association). He was running for the Presidency of the CHFA in Vancouver, BC during the annual health food convention in 1991. As the editor of the *Canadian Health & Nutrition Business Journal*, I had the opportunity to interview him and learn about his Yin-Yang drink that he was introducing to the public through health food stores.

Dr. Fann confirms that unfortunately there is not enough scientific evidence about Kombucha. He says, "we know that vinegar is healthy," implying that, much like Kombucha, science has not tested vinegar for its healthful properties. Convinced of the health bestowing agents in Kombucha, Dr. Fann created a new kind of soft drink that is a product of Kombucha fermentation. According to Dr. Fann, the living culture in the Kombucha mushroom is different from, for instance, *acidophilus* that stays in the intestines.

Instead, the Kombucha culture, says he, "produces healthful substances on fermenting." He claims that the culture does not as such become part of the intestinal flora. Yet this would not necessarily deny its usefulness to the intestinal flora. *Lactobacillus bulgaricus*, for instance, is a so-called "transient visitor" to our intestines and is known to be very beneficial to digestion, so is *Streptococcus thermophilus*. Both strains are not normally resident in the human intestines, but are used in yogurt making and are known to benefit our health by staying in the intestines for up to two weeks or more.

To obtain a durable health drink with a long shelf life, Dr. Fann pasteurizes his Yin-Yang drink. This process he admits kills the living Kombucha culture, but leaves behind the essence of its ingredients. Dr. Fann disagrees that the Kombucha must be prepared using green or black tea. Instead he employs herbal teas that result, he says, "in a drink that is free of caffeine." Again, contrary to the history of this folk remedy, Fann uses honey or grape juice as a sweet food source for his Yin-Yang drink. Also, to obtain a more palatable taste that is not too sour, he ferments the Yin-Yang drink for only a short period of time.

Dr. Fann tells me that when he has completed his research, he plans to write a book on Kombucha that will show scientific proof of the benefits of the health drink that is sweeping the world.

Help the Medicine Go Down

In case you love the tea ceremony at home but find your tea has gone sour, you can soften the taste of your finished Kombucha drink by simply adding water. Of course, Kombucha tea lends itself to mixing with other beverages as well. So if you are looking to experiment with your home brew, try mixing 1/2 Kombucha tea with 1/2 apple juice. Children will enjoy that blend. To soften the flavor you can also mix it with green tea or raspberry tea. Then, there are berry syrups to try out. Do you want to be really adventurous? Throw a Kombucha party and have guests try out various mixes and do-it-yourself recipes.

Some Kombucha experts suggest flavor improvements by fermenting in herbal teas such as raspberry leaves, blackberry leaves or dandelions. I would again caution the adventurous to first familiarize themselves with the medicinal effects of the herbal tea with which they wish to experiment. Another caution is that herbal teas should be preferably from herbs that are homegrown because of the freshness factor. So before you embark on the herbal Kombucha road, study a good book on herbs, take a course from a herbalist, or leave it to the experts and stick to black teas.

To help the medicine go down, here is my recipe for Kombucha champagne: prepare your Kombucha tea with Orange Pekoe, using 1/2 cup of refined white sugar per liter of tea and ferment in a dark, airy place preferably high up on a shelf in the basement near the air vent for a total of eight days. Pour into a champagne glass, straining it through a cotton sieve. Watch the bubbles rise. Drink on the spot. Every time I do it, it tastes just like champagne.

A Viable Vinegar

The best champagne can turn into vinegar if fermented too long. You may have accidentally discovered Kombucha vinegar this way. Your Kombucha tea will turn into a viable vinegar by letting it ferment for fifteen days or by leaving it for a longer time in the refrigerator. Remember the longer it is left, the more vinegary it will taste. You may use it like any other vinegar.

How Much and When to Drink Kombucha

You may want to consult your health care practitioner. As a rough yardstick, my wife and I drink 1/2 cup (125 ml) on an empty stomach early in the morning and again 1/2 cup before bed at night. We are planning to increase our intake to 1 cup (250 ml) in the morning and 1 cup in the evening. However, that is only for us and not a guideline for others. The answer to this question varies depending on the expert being consulted. Recommendations vary from 1/2 cup on an empty stomach or 1/4 cup before each meal to 1/8 liter after the main meal of the day. Within reason, I would suggest that is not crucial when and how much Kombucha you drink, as long as you do it regularly before taking a break in your routine.

Any Unwanted Side Effects to Kombucha?

Harald Tietze would probably say that there are definitely no unwanted side effects. He apparently drank up to three liters of Kombucha every day for six weeks and felt great. Hobbs quotes a mushroom cultivator in Washington State who is dead against Kombucha because he fears contamination of the culture by pathogenic microbes. Is it possible? There is no literature to support this fear.

If properly handled, there should not be any unwanted side effects or intolerance of Kombucha tea. Diabetics obviously should carefully watch the fermentation process to monitor sugar content. If reason and logic prevail in the fermentation and you are following all the recommendations, there should not be any problem. When in doubt, always check with your health care provider.

Otherwise, you are on your own. I report the information and it is up to you to decide on the evidence before you whether you deem Kombucha safe. Betsy Pryor tells us that both the FDA and the State of California have inspected her Kombucha batches several times and found them completely safe. Probably millions of people the world over safely drink Kombucha and other fermented drinks and foods. The culture contains its own antibacterial (acidic) weaponry against harmful bacteria. Even Hobbs agrees that with proper and careful preparation the Kombucha culture should be safe and without unwanted side effects. Kombucha can be used effectively for several ailments as long as you start slowly and do not try to cure any major diseases with it.

Is Kombucha a Miracle Healer?

The answer is no, though my first response to this question is yes. There are so many reports that Kombucha tea has restored health and cured ailments of various kinds, that it seems like a cure-all. While not a cure-all, testimonials clearly and overwhelmingly state that Kombucha tea does rejuvenate your body.

Kombucha farmer Betsy Pryor was converted from a "Saul to a Paul." During a recent seminar she said, "I thought it was snake oil. I really want to be honest about that. It did too many things. I didn't think it was possible for any one thing to affect things from arthritis to T-cells to psoriasis. I just didn't believe this." In time, her cynical view changed. Sklenar's impeccable research in Germany and the Russian investigations convinced her that it can help the body to heal itself through its balancing mechanism triggered by the glucuronic acid. However, she is the first to admit that "it isn't a cure for anything."

Regardless, in time, scientific tests will be carried out that will confirm what we already know - Kombucha works explainable miracles. As previously mentioned, homeopathic doctors and other practitioners have used these established treatments successfully on their patients. So Kombucha cannot be dismissed as simply snake oil.

The Future of Kombucha

The next millennium may see the necessity of feeding its advancing billions on simpler fare such as Kombucha tea. As our world continues to exhaust its resources, rediscovery of ancient methods of food preparation will become valuable. For example, fermented beverages such as Kombucha tea are becoming accepted into mainstream notions of healthy drinks. Although questions still need to be answered regarding the healing properties of Kombucha tea, there are two aspects of the tea that should be remembered. Firstly, testimonials clearly indicate that Kombucha tea aids digestion and detoxification, increasing overall energy. Secondly, Kombucha provides an inexpensive and delicious alternative to the high sugar and preservative content in alcoholic or carbonated beverages.

With Kombucha tea in hand, you'll be able to face the future with enthusiasm and cheer.

Cheers - Salute - Kan Bei - Nas Drovje - Cin Cin - Prost!

Commonly Asked Questions:

Q: Where do I get a Kombucha mushroom?
A: Check in the Resources section for professional suppliers or see your local natural food dealer or natural health publication for a reliable source. Only buy or accept Kombuchas from someone you trust. It is important to have a healthy and viable Kombucha for breeding "babies" and making the tea.

Q: How should I store the Kombucha until I use it?
A: Float it in a cup of sweetened tea in a glass container inside the refrigerator. It will store well like that for up to three months.

Q: Can I store or ferment a Kombucha in plastic or metal?
A: According to reliable research, a Kombucha leaches possibly harmful compounds from plastics (hydrocarbons) or metal (iron, steel, aluminum) and incorporates them into its structure, passing the compounds on to its babies and the tea. With this in mind, avoid plastic and metal utensils and containers, and lead crystal bowls for handling or fermenting Kombucha. Use ordinary or Pyrex glass!

Q: Can I brew Kombucha tea without refined white sugar?
A: My advice is to stick to the recipe. For beginners, I recommend making the tea with sugar, according to the instructions in Part Three - Tea Ceremony. Some people try molasses, dark sugars or honey to create their Kombucha tea. Experiment at your own risk if you are an advanced user. But, remember that the sugar is not for you, it is there to feed the yeast that would die without it. If you want to avoid sugar, allow a longer fermentation period (at least 14 days) or use a little less sugar.

Q: How will I know if my tea turned out right?
A: If you followed my recipe to the letter, nothing should have gone wrong. After a successful brew, a baby should be formed. It can be on top of the mother or, because the mother sank, on top of the tea.

Q: My Kombucha sank to the bottom of the bowl, is it dead?
A: If there is less oxygen in the Kombucha mother, it may sink to the bottom. As long as it produced a healthy baby, all should be well.

Q: Can I cut a Kombucha in half and make two batches?
A: Yes, you can even cut it in thirds and make three batches. As long as you do everything according to the instructions, you will be fine.

Q: My Kombucha is very thin, is this normal?
A: Yes. Kombuchas come in all shapes and sizes and under colder conditions will produce thinner babies, that are viable. To avoid this, place the fermentation into a warmer environment (22°-30° Celsius is optimal) or try adding more sugar to increase growth during the winter months.

Q: My Kombucha is covered in mold, what should I do?
A: The safest thing to do is throw it out and start afresh. Fruit flies and other contaminants may have got in your mixture. For this reason, keep your Kombucha properly sealed, but able to breathe, and away from plants, fruits, vegetables, compost or garbage. Perhaps the Kombucha you received was contaminated. I repeat, "when in doubt, throw it out!"

Q: If a Kombucha becomes dried out, can I still use it?
A: If it was not in contact with contaminants (food particles, fruit flies, metals, plastics), you should be able to revive it. Simply rinse the mushroom with Kombucha tea or apple cider vinegar. Let it soak for 15 minutes in the tea or vinegar. Then, proceed with a new batch of tea according to my instructions, adding a bit of the tea or vinegar you used for rinsing the Kombucha. If your new tea does not turn out, the Kombucha may be dead. Throw it out and get another.

Q: Can Kombucha tea make a mushroom all on its own?
A: Well, it can if you left the Kombucha tea sitting in a warm spot for an extended period of time. To prevent your Kombucha tea from fermenting further and making a mushroom, put it in the fridge.

Q: Should I use a glass bowl, jar or cylinder for making the tea?
A: For the best fermenting conditions, ferment your tea in a glass bowl. Fermenting in a bowl results in a moderately sized Kombucha mushroom, while lasagna or casserole dishes result in a larger mushroom. Also, a bowl allows for more exposure to the tea mixture and to oxygen than jars and cylinders which are too narrow.

Q: Will Kombucha tea cure my Chronic Fatigue Syndrome?
A: Kombucha is not a cure for any disease. Rather, use Kombucha to augment your health regime of optimal nutrition, exercise, rest, and last but not least, spiritual nourishment. Kombucha tea aids digestion, improves metabolism and provides extra energy. For these reasons, it can be a benefit to anyone suffering from deficient health. However, if you suffer from a serious disease, you should consult your health care practitioner.

Q: Can Kombucha cure cancer?
A: No one can be sure whether or not Kombucha cures cancer, but several practitioners have reduced tumors with nothing other than Kombucha tea, notably the German physician Dr. Sklenar. Also, the noted medical scientist Dr. Johannes Kuhl takes notice of the cancer-fighting properties of lactic acid fermented products.

Q: What is lactic acid fermentation?
A: Lactic acid is an end product of carbohydrate (sugar) fermentation by friendly microorganisms. In Kombucha these organisms cause mainly L (+) lactic acid, the good acid. Breakdown of glycogen (glycolysis) causes lactic acid accumulation in active muscle tissues. Kombucha is not related to yogurt or kefir, but because lactic acid was first found in milk, it was named "lactic" from the Latin word "lac" for milk.

Q: Can I eat my Kombucha?
A: While eating a Kombucha is possible, it is not recommended. A Kombucha mushroom is hard to digest because of its cellulose content. My advice is to keep it alive to make more delicious healthful tea. Professional Kombucha extracts are sold in natural food stores, mainly for use by diabetics.

Q: Can I give Kombucha tea to my pet?
A: Yes, Kombucha can be given safely to your furry loved ones. As little as a tablespoon per day diluted in drinking water or food or, if preferred, administered by a small oral syringe will provide them with their daily dose. Large animals can be given twice that dosage.

Recommended Reading

Balch, James & Phyllis. 1990. *Prescription for Nutritional Healing*. Garden City Park, NY: Avery Publishing Group.

Levin, James & Natalie Cederquist. 1993. *Vibrant Living*. San Diego, CA: GLO, Inc.

Weiss, Rudolf Fritz. 1988. *Herbal Medicine*. Beaconsfield, England: Beaconsfield Publishers.

Resources

Alive Academy of Nutrition
7436 Fraser Park Drive
Burnaby BC V5J 5B9
604-435-1919
Fax: 604-435-4888

Coastal Mountain College of Healing Arts Inc
1745 West 4th Avenue
Vancouver BC V6J 1M2
604-734-4596
Fax: 604-734-4597

Wild Rose College of Natural Healing
400 - 1228 Kensington Road NW
Calgary AB T2N 3P5
403-270-0936
Fax: 403-283-0799

For Bottled Kombucha Tea and Extracts:

ProNatura Inc
6211 - A West Howard Street
Niles IL 60714
708-588-0900
Fax: 708-588-0918

Béland Foods
Box 1911
Sechelt BC V0N 3A0
604-886-0766
Fax: 604-253-0439

Pro-Organics
3454 Lougheed Highway
Vancouver BC V5M 2A4
604-253-6549
Fax: 604-253-0439

Flora Distributing Ltd
7400 Fraser Park Drive
Burnaby BC V5J 5B9
604-436-6000
Fax: 604-436-6060

Purity Life Ltd
6 Commerce Crescent
Acton ON L7J 2X3
519-853-3511
800-930-9512
Fax: 519-853-4660
– or –
2975 Lake City Way
Burnaby BC V5A 2Z6
604-421-8931
800-665-8830
Fax: 604-421-8951

Yin-Yang Natural Products
37 Kingswood Road
Toronto ON M4E 3N4
416-691-3038
Fax: 416-691-5760

Capital Santé
1670 Du Ruisseau
Ste-Adèle PQ J0R 1L0
514-229-7808
Fax: 514-229-3064

For Kombucha Mushrooms:

Klaus Kaufmann
9566 Willowleaf Place
Burnaby BC V5A 4A5
Fax: 604-421-3610

B & B Farms
RR #3 273 Hunter Road
Niagara-on-the-Lake ON L0S 1J0
Phone or Fax: 905-262-5075

Bibliography

Ahmadjian, Vernon & Surinda Paracer. 1986. *Symbiosis*. Hanover, NH: University Press.

Chaitow, Leon & Natasha Trenves. 1990. *ProBiotics*. Wellingborough, England: Thorsons.

Fasching, Rosina. 1985, 1989. *Le champignon de longue vie combucha*. Steyr, Austria: W. Ennsthaler.

Fasching, Rosina. 1987. *Tea Fungus Kombucha*. Steyr, Austria: W. Ennsthaler.

Fischer, William L. 1987. *How to Fight Cancer & Win*. Vancouver, BC: Alive Books.

Frank, Günther W. 1991. *Kombucha - Das Teepilz-Getränk*. Steyr, Austria: W. Ennsthaler.

Golz, Helmut. 1990, 1992. *Kombucha - Ein altes Teeheilmittel*. München, Germany: Ariston Verlag.

Haard, Richard & Karen. 1980. *Poisonous & Hallucinogenic Mushrooms*. Seattle, WA: Homestead Book Co.

Haard, Richard & Karen. 1980. *Foraging for Edible Wild Mushrooms*. Seattle, WA: Homestead Book Co.

Harnisch, Günther. 1991. *Kombucha, Geballte Heilkraft aus der Natur*. Germany: Turm, B.

Hobbs, Christopher. 1995. *Kombucha: Tea Mushroom - The Essential Guide*. Santa Cruz, CA: Botanica Press.

Hobbs, Christopher. 1986, 1995. *Medicinal Mushrooms*. Santa Cruz, CA: Botanica Press.

Horizon. "Sex Under Siege." Produced by Deborah Cadbury. Edited by Jana Bennett. 50 min. BBC Science Features, 1993. Videocassette. (Available from CBC Educational Sales: 416-205-6384)

Pryor, Betsy & Sanford Holst. 1995. *Kombucha Phenomenon*. Sherman Oaks, CA: Sierra Sunrise Books.

Read, Clark P. 1970. *Parasitism and Symbiology*. New York, NY: Ronald Press.

Rossmoore, Harold W. 1976. *The Microbes, Our Unseen Friends*. Detroit, MI: Wayne State University Press.

Stevenson, Greta. 1970. *The Biology of Fungi, Bacteria and Viruses*. New York, NY: American Elsevier Publishing.

Tietze, Harald W. 1994. *Kombucha-The Miracle Fungus*. Bermagui South, NSW, Australia: Gateway Books.

Index

A

B

C

D

E F

G H

I K

L M

N O

P

R S

T U

V W Y

About the Author

Klaus Kaufmann is mainly self-taught. Historical events of World War II and the turmoil following denied him the privilege of completing university. Yet his thirst for knowledge remained unquenchable. Klaus has been studying natural healing properties for many years. His search for a more natural lifestyle took him all over the globe. Following a photo safari to Africa, he decided to live in Southern Africa for some years. Then, he took his wife to the equatorial reaches, spending a year on a teaching permit in Kuala Lumpur, Malaysia. During 1977, the Kaufmanns moved to White Rock, BC to participate in miniature horse breeding. Klaus had started the first such horse farm in Canada several years earlier with friends.

In the years that followed, his interest in writing blossomed alongside his growing interest in all matters scientific. Following the study of English literature and creative writing at university, his professor appointed Klaus editor of *CONTACT*, a Canadian Writers Guild publication. Under his editorship, the publication expanded from a simple newsletter to a magazine. When Klaus left, the publication was popular in book shops and read at universities across Canada and in England. At a live performance in Toronto, "Jazz and Poetry" selected Klaus' poetry for a public reading. Before being published under his own name, Klaus worked as a ghost writer.

His enormously popular best-seller, *Silica - The Forgotten Nutrient*, now in its second edition, was quickly followed by *The Joy of Juice Fasting* that also made the best-seller list. During 1991, Klaus became concerned with the problem of mercury toxicity and wrote *Eliminating Poison in Your Mouth*. His 1993 best-seller, *Silica - The Amazing Gel*, is the companion volume to the first silica book. Apart from his writing, Klaus is researching and completing a Doctor of Science degree. Klaus and his wife Gabryelle live at Burnaby Mountain in British Columbia.

If you use Kombucha tea remedially on your pets and are successful, I would appreciate hearing from you.
Please mail your report to:

Klaus Kaufmann
c/o Alive Books
7436 Fraser Park Drive
Burnaby BC V5J 5B9 Canada
Fax: 604-435-4888

Other titles by Klaus Kaufmann

Silica - The Forgotten Nutrient
Healthy Skin, Shiny Hair, Strong Bones, Beautiful Nails - A guide to the vital role of organic vegetal silica in nutrition, health, longevity and medicine.
Klaus Kaufmann, 1990, 1993, 128 pp softcover

Silica - The Amazing Gel
An essential mineral for radiant health, recovery and rejuvenation.
Klaus Kaufmann, 1993, 1995, 159 pp softcover

The Joy of Juice Fasting
For Health & Cleansing & Weight Loss.
Klaus Kaufmann, 1990, 114 pp softcover

Eliminating Poison in Your Mouth
Overcoming Mercury Amalgam Toxicity.
Klaus Kaufmann, 1991, 44 pp softcover

Other titles by Alive Books

Return to the Joy of Health
Natural medicine and alternative treatments for all your health complaints.
Dr. Zoltan Rona, 408 pp softcover

A Diet for All Reasons
A nutrition guide and recipe collection for beginner vegetarians.
Paulette Eisen, 176 pp softcover, special bound

The Breuss Cancer Cure
Advice for prevention and natural treatment of cancer, leukemia and other seemingly incurable diseases.
Rudolf Breuss (Translated from German), 112pp softcover

Fats That Heal Fats That Kill
The complete guide to fats, oils, cholesterol and human health.
Udo Erasmus, 480 pp softcover

Healing with Herbal Juices
A practical guide to herbal juice therapy: nature's preventative medicine.
Siegfried Gursche, 256 pp softcover

Making Sauerkraut and Pickled Vegetables at Home
The original lactic acid fermentation method.
Annelies Schoeneck, 80 pp softcover

Devil's Claw Root and Other Natural Remedies for Arthritis
A herbal remedy that has helped free thousands of arthritis sufferers from crippling pain.
Rachel Carston (Revised by Klaus Kaufmann), 128 pp softcover

Allergies: Disease in Disguise
How to heal your allergic condition permanently and naturally.
Carolee Bateson-Koch DC ND, 224 pp softcover

International Health News Yearbook (Annual)
The latest, most important discoveries in nutrition, health and medicine.
Hans Larsen, 96 pp softcover

All books are available at your local health food store, bookstore or from
Alive Books, PO Box 80055, Burnaby BC V5H 3X1